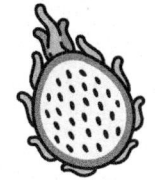
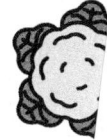

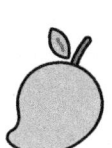
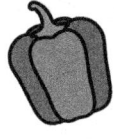
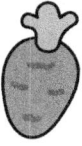

The Heart Healthy Meal Prep Cookbook for Beginners

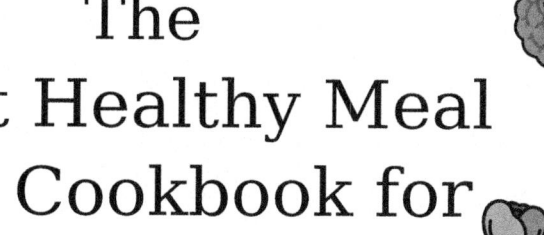
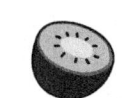
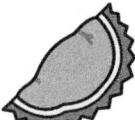

This book of:

....

....

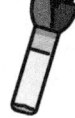
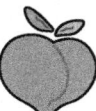
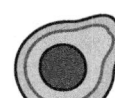
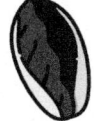
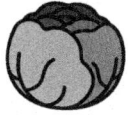
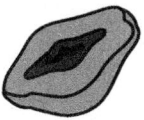

Table of contents

PART 1 — Main dish

PART 2 — Dessert

PART 3 — Soup

PART 4 — Salad

PART 5 — Dink

PART 6 — Dressings, Sauces and Jams

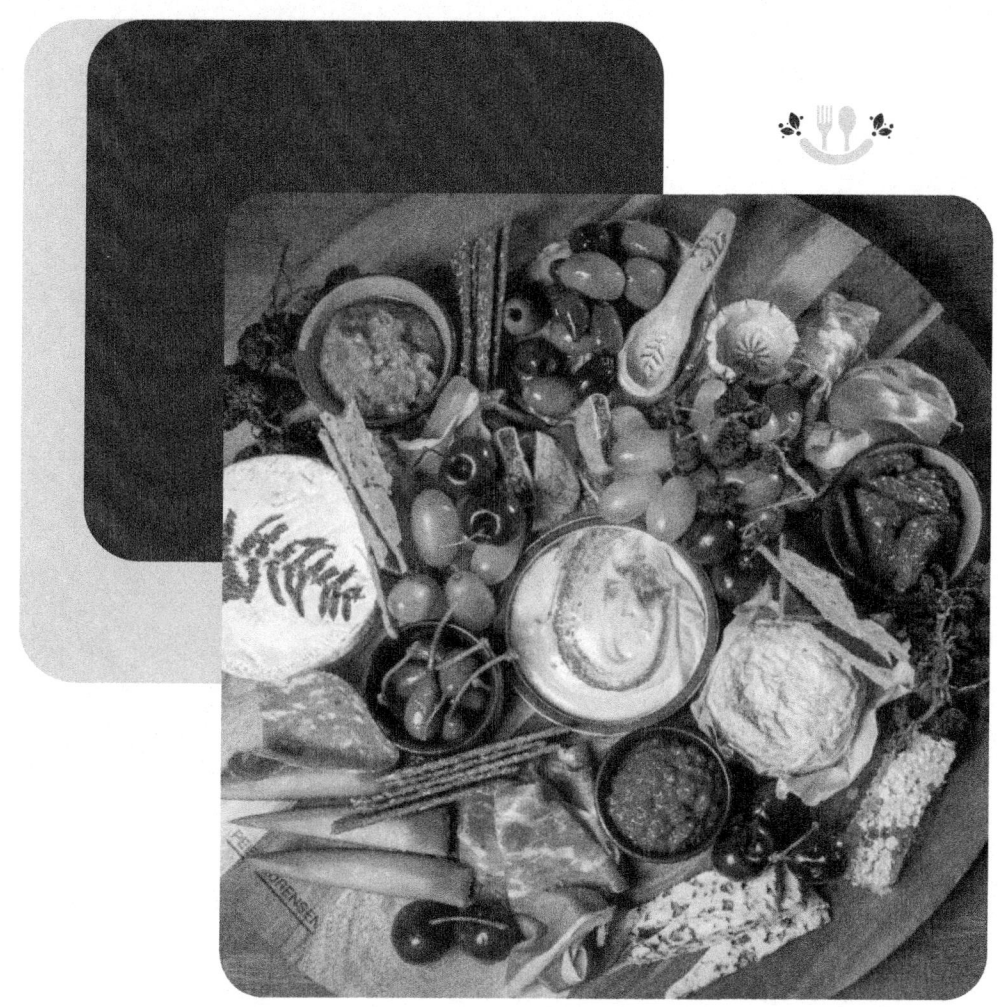

Main dish

A main dish, also known as an entrée or main course, is the central or primary part of a meal around which the other courses are built. This dish is typically the most substantial, hearty, and filling component of a meal. In many culinary traditions, the main dish focuses on a key source of protein such as meat, fish, or a substantial vegetarian alternative like tofu or legumes. It is often accompanied by a combination of vegetables, grains, or starches that complement the flavors and textures of the primary ingredient. The main dish is designed to satisfy hunger and provide the bulk of nutritional intake from the meal.

Smoked Salmon with Beurre Blanc and Soft Poached Egg

SERVES 4

For the Beurre Blanc
- ½ cup dry white wine
- ½ cup white wine vinegar
- 4 tbsp diced shallots
- 2/3 cup cream
- ½ tsp salt
- ¼ tsp white pepper
- 2 cups unsalted butter, cut into cubes and chilled

For the Eggs
- 4 eggs
- Pinch of salt

To serve
- 200 g cold smoked salmon
- 2 radishes, thinly sliced
- ½ Lebanese cucumber, finely diced
- Micro herbs
- Edible flowers

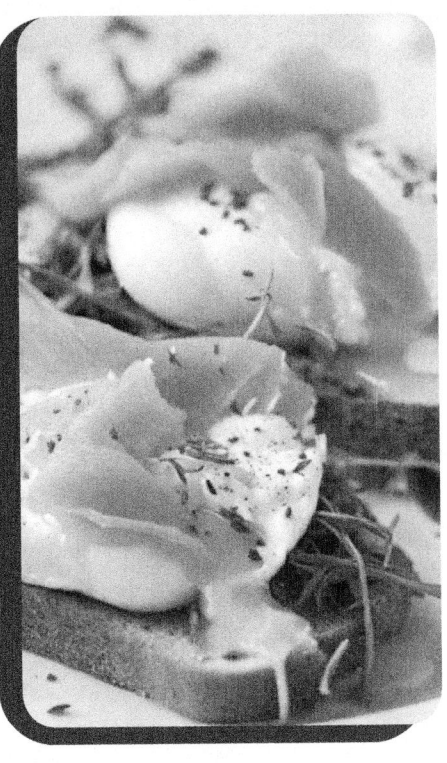

DIRECTIONS

1. Make Beurre Blanc by adding wine, vinegar and shallots to a small saucepan over medium heat. Bring to the boil and boil until the liquid has reduced to 2 to 3 tablespoons. Add cream, salt and pepper and boil for 1 minute, then reduce heat to low and add butter a few cubes at a time, whisking constantly. The butter should have completely melted before adding more. Remove from the heat and pour through a sieve to separate the shallot. Set aside.
2. Fill a large saucepan with water and place over medium heat. Bring water to a simmer and toss in salt. Crack eggs, one at a time, into a cup. Gently pour eggs into the water. Cook eggs for 2 minutes, then remove from the water using a slotted spoon. Place on a paper-towel lined plate and set aside.
3. To serve, add an egg yolk to each serving bowl. Spoon some of the beurre blanc into bowls, then place smoked salmon around the edges. Arrange radish slices, cucumber, edible flowers and micro herbs and serve.

Best Ever Potato Croquettes

SERVES 4

- 700 g Dutch Cream potatoes
- 3 eggs, divided
- 3 cloves garlic, minced
- ½ cup grated parmesan
- 1 tbsp flat leaf parsley, finely chopped
- Salt, to taste
- Freshly ground black pepper, to taste
- ¼ cup plain flour
- 1 tbsp water
- ¾ cup breadcrumbs
- 3 tbsp olive oil

DIRECTIONS

1. Make Beurre Blanc by adding wine, vinegar and shallots to a small saucepan over medium heat. Bring to the boil and boil until the liquid has reduced to 2 to 3 tablespoons. Add cream, salt and pepper and boil for 1 minute, then reduce heat to low and add butter a few cubes at a time, whisking constantly. The butter should have completely melted before adding more. Remove from the heat and pour through a sieve to separate the shallot. Set aside.
2. Fill a large saucepan with water and place over medium heat. Bring water to a simmer and toss in salt. Crack eggs, one at a time, into a cup. Gently pour eggs into the water. Cook eggs for 2 minutes, then remove from the water using a slotted spoon. Place on a paper-towel lined plate and set aside.
3. To serve, add an egg yolk to each serving bowl. Spoon some of the beurre blanc into bowls, then place smoked salmon around the edges. Arrange radish slices, cucumber, edible flowers and micro herbs and serve.

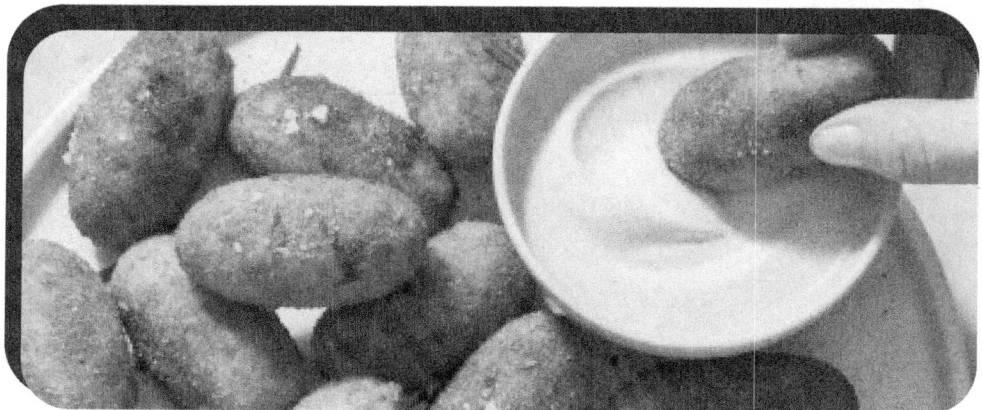

Pea Pods with Green Pesto

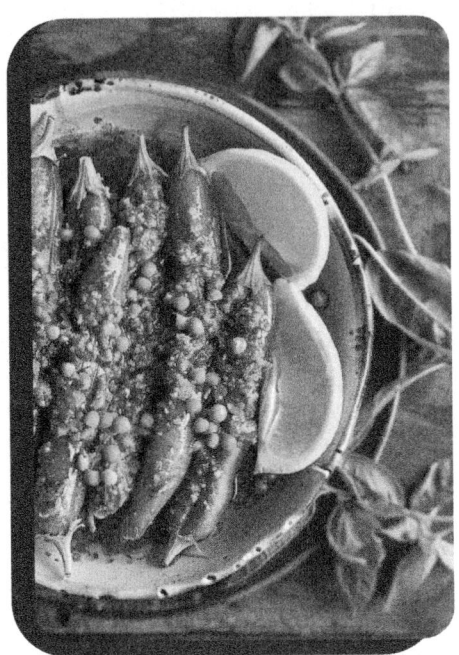

SERVES 2

- ¾ cup walnuts, chopped and divided
- 2 cloves garlic
- 1 ½ cups flat leaf parsley
- ½ cup coriander leaves
- 2 tsp lemon juice
- 1/3 cup olive oil
- 1 cup sugar snap or snow peas, divided
- Lemon slices to serve

DIRECTIONS

1. Add garlic, parsley, coriander, lemon juice and olive oil to a food processor with ½ cup walnuts. Blitz on high speed until all ingredients are combined.
2. Serve topped with remaining ¼ cup walnuts, lemon slices and fresh snow or sugar snap peas.

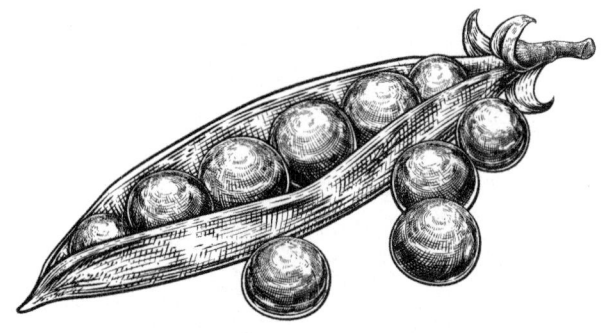

Oysters with Fresh Wasabi Cream

MAKES 24 OYSTERS

- 24 oysters
- 2 tbsp grated fresh wasabi (alternatively horseradish)
- 2 tsp red wine vinegar
- 80 g crème fraiche
- ¼ tsp sea salt
- 50 g Petuna Ocean Trout Caviar
- Freshly ground black pepper
- 500g rock salt, for plating

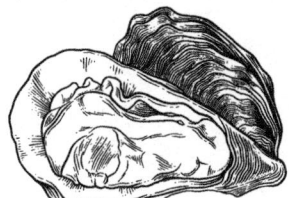
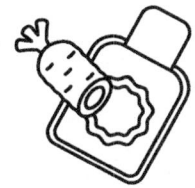

DIRECTIONS

1. Add wasabi, vinegar, crème fraiche and salt to a bowl. Stir to combine and taste for seasoning. Pour into a small serving bowl and garnish with a grind of fresh pepper and grated wasabi optional.
2. Place the bowl of wasabi cream on a platter along with a spoon. Cover the base of the platter with rock salt. Arrange oysters on top and scatter with caviar. Serve immediately.

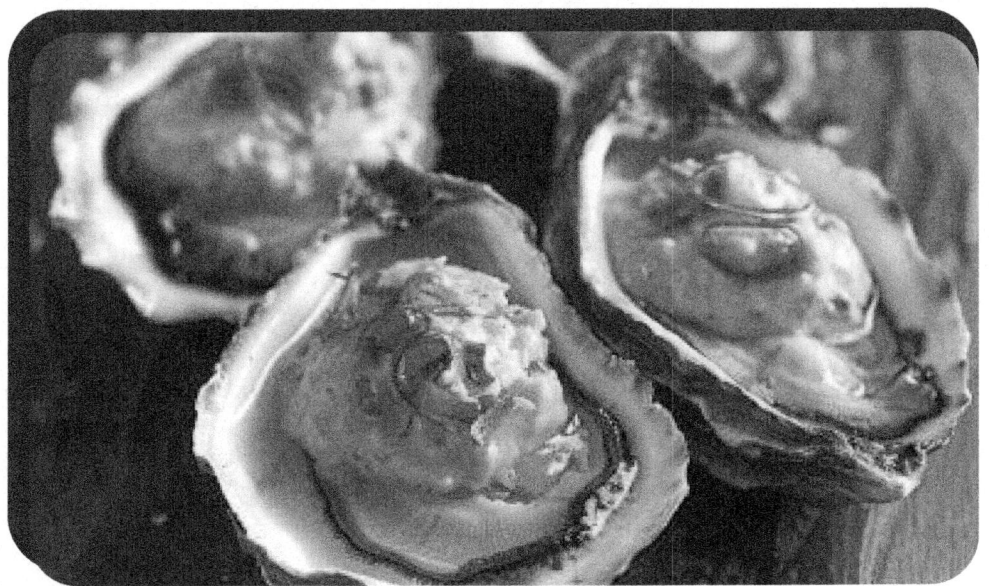

Whole Stuffed Mushrooms

SERVES 4

- 16 whole mushrooms, about 7 centimetres in diameter
- 4 tbsp olive oil, divided
- ¼ cup brown onion, finely diced
- 2 cloves garlic, minced
- 4 tbsp parsley, finely chopped, divided
- 75 g baby spinach leaves
- ½ cup breadcrumbs
- ¼ cup Parmesan, grated
- 1 tsp oregano, finely chopped
- Salt
- Freshly ground black pepper
- 2 tbsp tomato paste

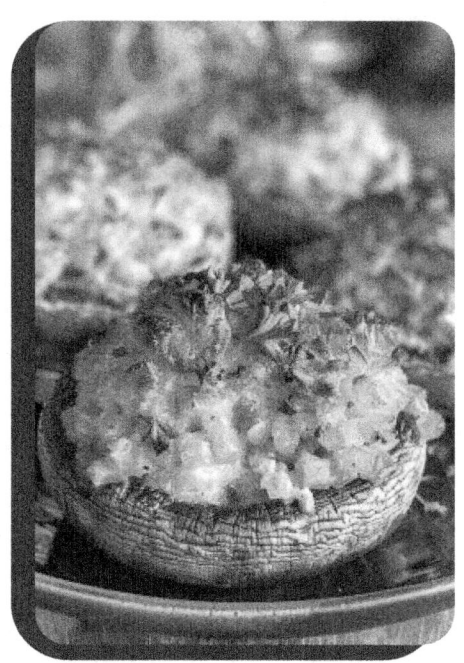

DIRECTIONS

1. Preheat oven to 180C.
2. Wipe mushrooms with paper towel to remove any excess dirt. Remove stems from mushrooms and finely chop.
3. Heat a non-stick frying pan over medium heat and add 2 tablespoons olive oil. Add onion, garlic, chopped mushroom stems, and 3 tablespoons parsley to the frying pan. Cook for 2 minutes, then add spinach and reduce heat to low. Cook, covered, stirring occasionally for a further 5 minutes, or until the spinach has wilted and the other ingredients are soft.
4. Transfer mixture to a bowl and add breadcrumbs, parmesan, oregano and salt and pepper to taste.
5. Arrange mushrooms in a lined baking tray. Spoon a little tomato paste on top of each mushroom, then stuff the mixture into the mushrooms, pushing down with a spoon to fill them well.
6. Drizzle remaining olive oil over the mushrooms and cover the baking tray with foil. Cook in oven for 20 minutes, then remove the foil and cook for a further 10 minutes, or until the mushrooms are golden brown.
7. Garnish with remaining parsley and serve while hot.

Brie with Beetroot Pachadi, Pear Jus and Pine Nuts

SERVES 4

For the Beetroot Pachadi
- 1 tbsp olive oil
- 2 tbsp raw peanuts, chopped
- 1 clove garlic
- 1 green chilli
- 1 red chilli
- 1 tbsp coriander leaves
- ½ tsp cumin seeds
- 1 cup beetroot, finely diced
- Salt
- Lemon juice

For the Pear Jus
- 6 pears, peeled and diced
- 1 cup vegetable stock
- 1 tsp ginger, minced
- 1 shallot, thinly sliced

To serve
- ½ cup pine nuts
- 200 g brie
- Pumpernickel, thickly sliced
- Smoked paprika, to garnish

DIRECTIONS

1. Heat oil in a frying pan over high heat. Add peanuts and fry until golden and aromatic, then add garlic, red and green chilli, cumin seeds, and coriander leaves. Fry until the leaves become crisp, then remove from pan and set aside to cool. Add beetroot to the pan and cook for 5 minutes, or until it is slightly tender. Remove from heat and set aside to cool.
2. When ingredients have cooled, blend with a stick blender, leaving some chunks of beetroot. Taste and add lemon juice if desired. Refrigerate until ready to serve.
3. Meanwhile make the pear jus by adding all ingredients to a saucepan. Bring to the boil, then reduce heat and leave to simmer until the sauce has reduced by half. Remove from heat and set aside to cool. When cool, puree with a stick blender until smooth. Refrigerate until ready to serve.
4. Preheat oven to 180C.
5. Heat a non-stick frying pan over medium-low heat. Add pine nuts and toast, stirring constantly until fragrant and golden. Transfer to a plate to stop them cooking and prevent burning.
6. Add thick slices of pumpernickel to a lined baking tray. Cut wedges of brie and lay on top of pumpernickel. Cook in the oven until the brie is starting to melt.
7. To serve, add pumpernickel and brie to serving plate, dollop some pear jus on the plate and add beetroot pachadi. Sprinkle with pine nuts and garnish with smoked paprika.

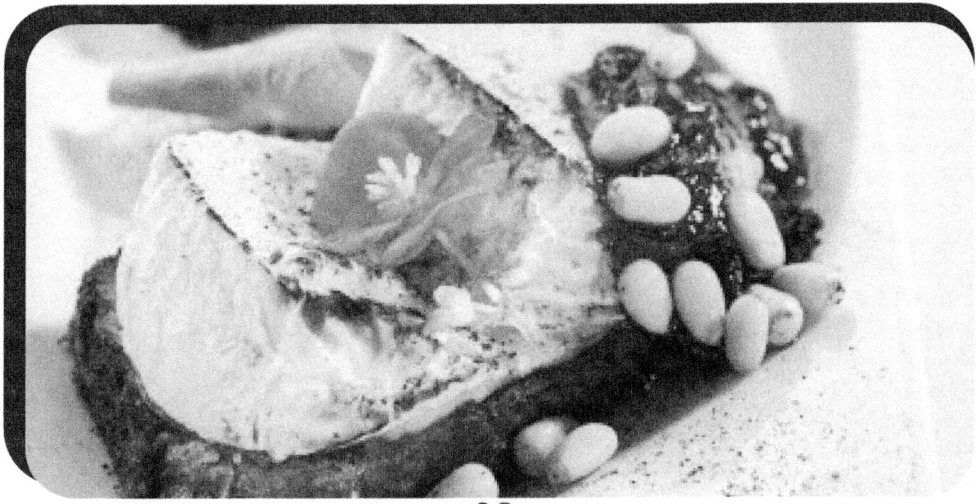

Oven Roasted Seasoned Greek Tomatoes

SERVES 6

- 500 g cherry tomatoes
- 4 tbsp olive oil
- 1 tsp cumin seeds
- 4 cloves garlic, minced
- 1 tsp dried thyme
- 1 tsp brown sugar
- Zest of 1 lemon, divided
- Salt
- Freshly ground black pepper
- 6 sprigs fresh oregano
- 500 g Greek yoghurt
- 1 tsp chilli flakes

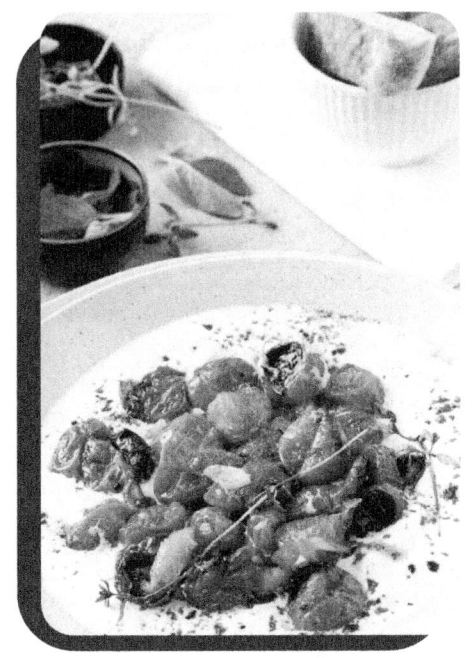

DIRECTIONS

1. Preheat oven to 220C.
2. Add tomatoes to a large bowl with olive oil, cumin seeds, garlic, thyme, brown sugar, half the lemon zest, salt and pepper. Toss to combine and then add to a baking tray. Scatter over oregano and cook in oven for 20 minutes.
3. Whisk remaining lemon zest with yoghurt and season with salt to taste.
4. To serve, add yoghurt to a large serving bowl and spoon tomatoes over the top. Garnish with chilli flakes and enjoy with bread.

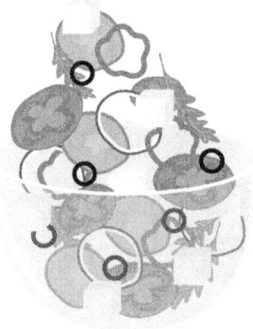
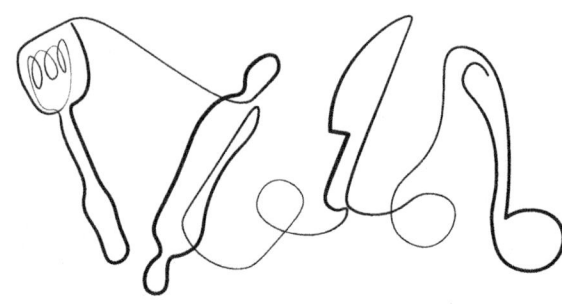

Quail with Balsamic Roasted Grapes

SERVES 6

- 6 quail
- 60 g butter, softened
- 600 g assorted grapes
- ¼ cup olive oil
- 2/3 cup white balsamic vinegar

DIRECTIONS

1. Preheat oven to 200C.
2. Rub quail all over with butter and season well with salt and pepper. Place quail on a baking tray lined with baking paper.
3. Place grapes on an oven tray and drizzle with olive oil and balsamic. Roast quail and grapes for 20 to 30 minutes or until the quail are golden and cooked through. Remove from oven and serve.

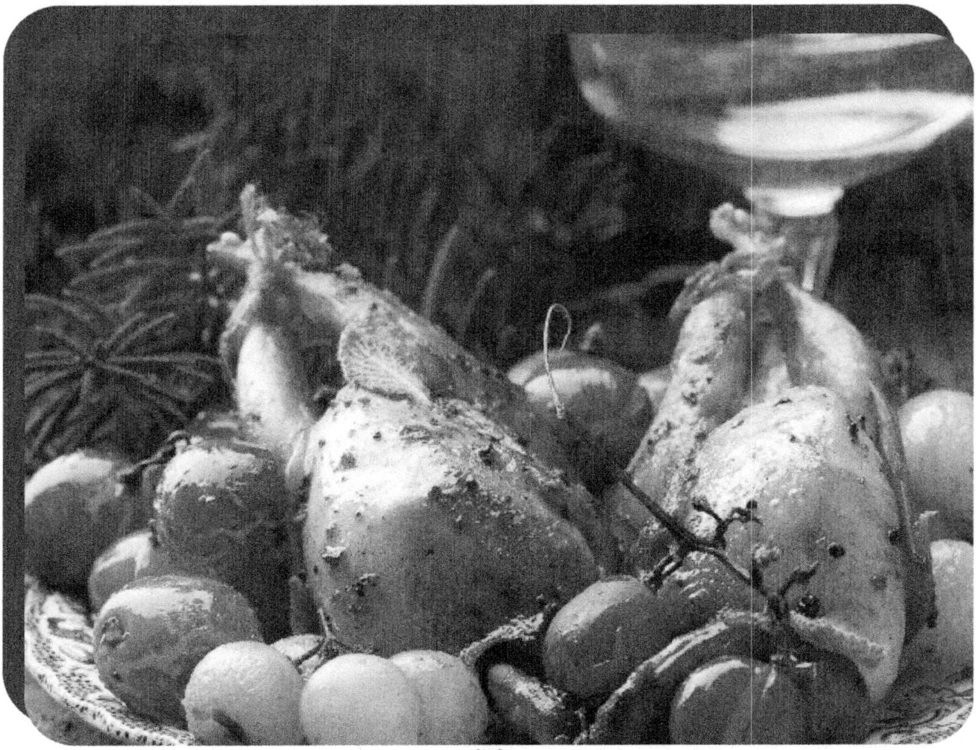

Roasted Stuffed Mushrooms

SERVES 4 AS A SNACK

- 16 cup mushrooms, stalks removed
- 50 g ham, diced
- 30 g sundried tomatoes, diced
- ¼ green capsicum, diced
- 40 g finely grated parmesan cheese

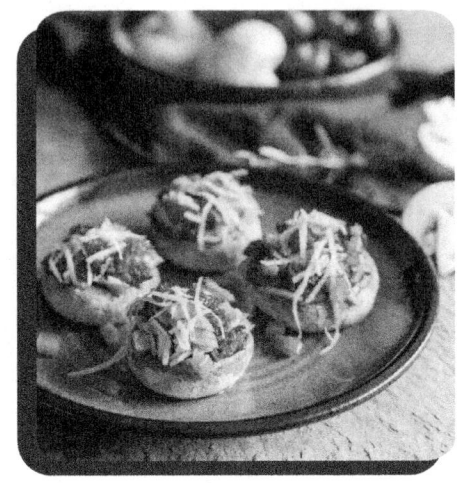

DIRECTIONS

1. Preheat oven to 200C.
2. Line a baking tray with baking paper and arrange mushrooms, with their caps down on the tray.
3. Combine ham, tomatoes, capsicum and parmesan in a bowl and stir. Season to taste.
4. Spoon mixture into mushrooms, then roast for 15 minutes, or until lightly browned.

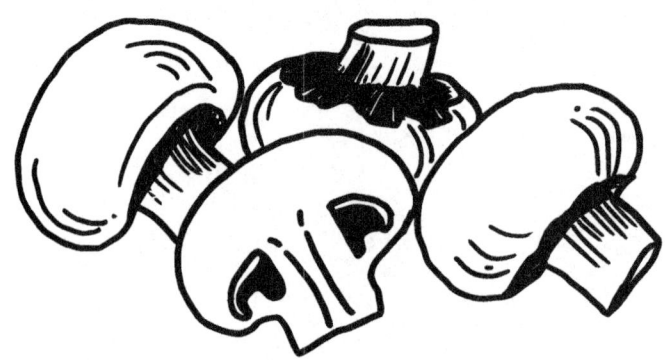

Iceberg Wedge Salad with Blue Cheese Dressing

SERVES 4

For the Salad
- 1 iceberg lettuce
- 4 rashers middle bacon, cooked and cooled
- 250 g cherry tomatoes, cut into wedges
- Salt
- Freshly ground black pepper

For the Blue Cheese Dressing
- 1 cup sour cream
- ½ cup mayonnaise
- 3 tbsp milk
- 3 tsp red wine vinegar
- 1 clove garlic, minced
- 120 g blue cheese
- 4 chives, chopped, reserve some chives for garnish

DIRECTIONS

1. Remove outer leaves from the iceberg lettuce, wash and cut in half, then cut each half into quartered wedges.
2. Prepare Blue Cheese Dressing by adding all ingredients to a mixing bowl and stirring to combine.
3. Place lettuce wedges onto serving plates and drizzle with Blue Cheese Dressing. Crumble over cooled bacon, and add tomatoes, then sprinkle with chives. Season with salt and pepper and serve.

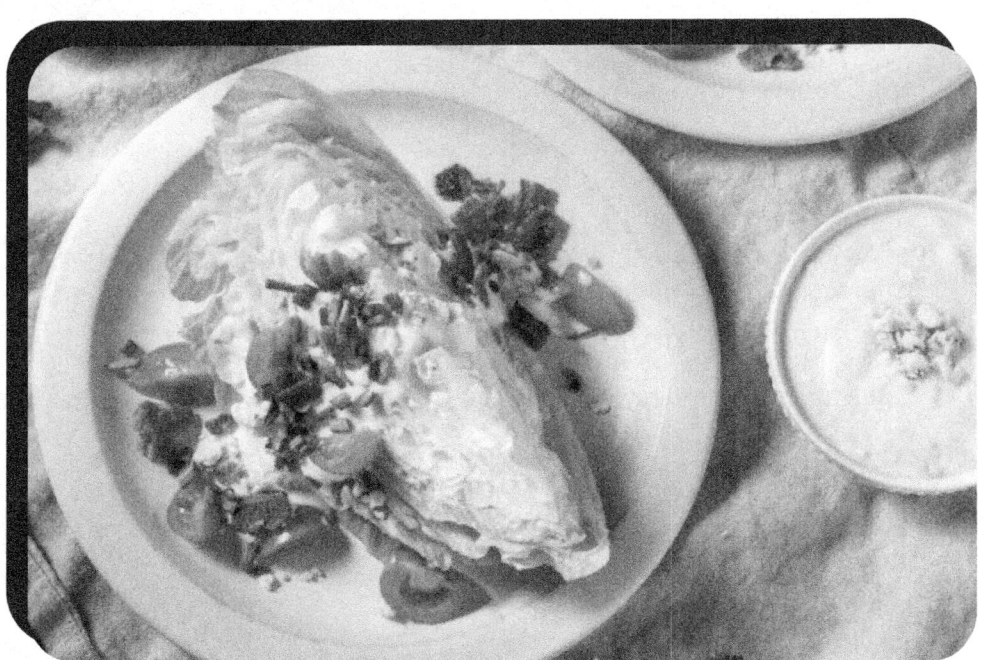

Cheesy Zucchini Pancakes

MAKES AROUND 12 PANCAKES

- 2 large zucchini, grated
- 2 spring onions, chopped
- 1 clove garlic, mined
- ½ cup plain flour
- 1 ½ tsp baking powder
- Pinch of salt
- Pinch of freshly ground black pepper
- ½ cup mozzarella cheese, grated
- ¼ cup parmesan cheese, grated
- 3 eggs, lightly whisked
- 2 tbsp olive oil, divided

To serve
- 1 cup sour cream
- ¼ bunch dill, finely chopped
- Lemon wedges

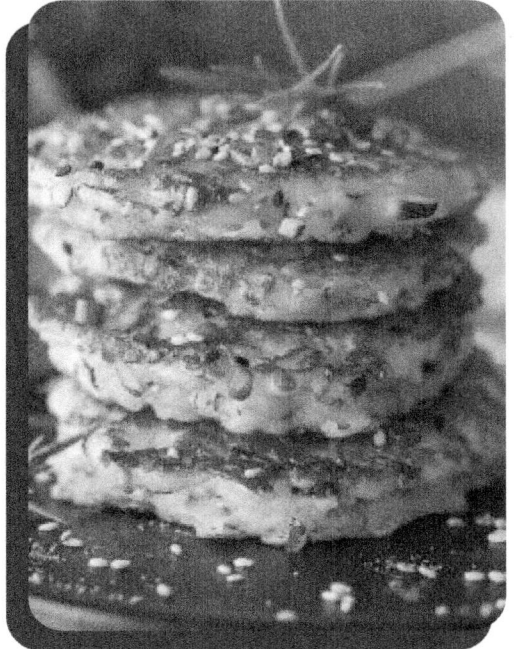

DIRECTIONS

1. Place grated zucchini in a clean tea towel and squeeze as much moisture from the grated zucchini as you can. Transfer to a bowl and add spring onions and garlic and stir to mix.
2. In a separate bowl add flour, baking powder, salt, pepper, mozzarella, and parmesan and stir to combine. Add eggs and zucchini, spring onion, and garlic and mix well.
3. Heat 1 tbsp olive oil in a frying pan over medium high heat. Add tablespoons of mixture to the hot pan and cook for 3-4 minutes per side. Repeat to use up all mixture.
4. Combine sour cream and dill in a small bowl and stir well. Serve pancakes warm with sour cream and lemon wedges.

Crispy Panko Prawns with Green Mango Noodle Salad

SERVES 4

- 100 g dried vermicelli noodles
- 50 g panko breadcrumbs
- 1 tbsp black sesame seeds, plus extra to serve
- 1 large free range egg white
- 1 kg whole jumbo green prawns
- 200g coconut oil
- 1 cucumber, julienned
- 1 large carrot, julienned
- ½ large green mango, julienned
- 4 spring onions, finely sliced
- ¼ cup basil leaves, torn
- ¼ cup mint leaves, torn, plus extra for garnish

For the dressing

- 3 birdseye chilli, roughly chopped
- 3 tbsp palm sugar, grated
- 5 tbsp lime juice
- 2 tbsp fish sauce

DIRECTIONS

1. Make dressing by blitzing the chilli and palm sugar in a small food processor until finely chopped. Add the lime juice and fish sauce and blitz to combine.
2. Peel and devein prawns, leaving the tails attached. Place in a bowl and add 3 tablespoons of dressing. Stir to combine and set aside to marinate.
3. Place noodles in a bowl and cover with boiling water. Set aside for 2 minutes or until the noodles have softened. Drain well, stir through half the remaining dressing, and set aside to cool.
4. Line a baking tray with baking paper.
5. Place egg white in a small bowl and lightly whisk. Place panko breadcrumbs and black sesame seeds in a separate bowl and mix to combine.
6. Using the tail to hold the prawns, dip half of each prawn into the egg white mix and then in the panko crumbs. Transfer to the lined baking tray.
7. Heat oil in a large frying pan over medium-high heat. Cook prawns in batches, for 1 minute each side or until golden, crisp and cooked through. Transfer to a plate lined with paper towel to drain.
8. Place the noodles, cucumber, carrot, green mango and herbs on a serving plate and toss to combine. Add prawns and drizzle with the remaining dressing. Sprinkle with black sesame seeds and herbs and serve.

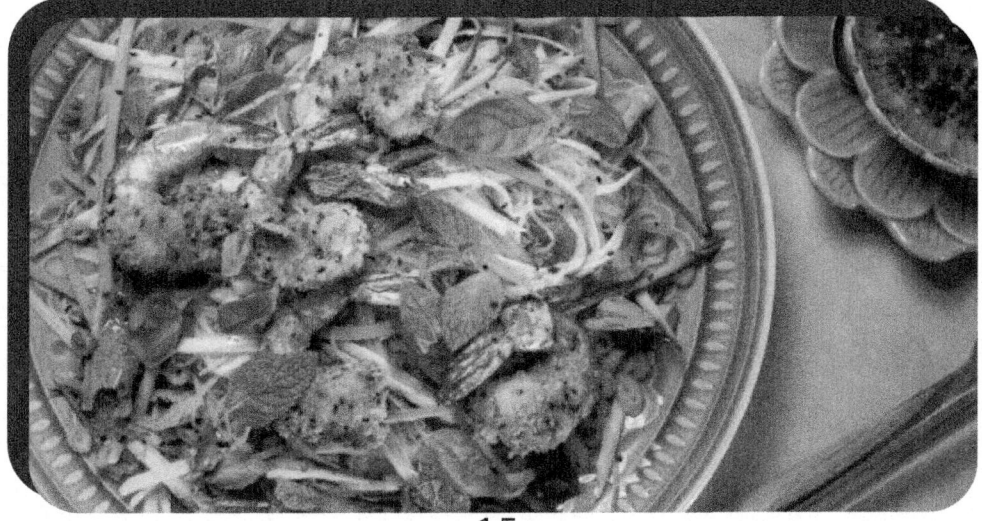

Roasted Pears with Roquefort, Walnuts and Honey

SERVES 4

- 4 beurre bosc pears
- 2 tsp brown sugar
- 80 g Roquefort, crumbled
- 2 tbsp honey
- 10 walnuts, roughly chopped
- 1 tbsp thyme leaves
- 1 tsp chilli flakes, plus extra for garnish

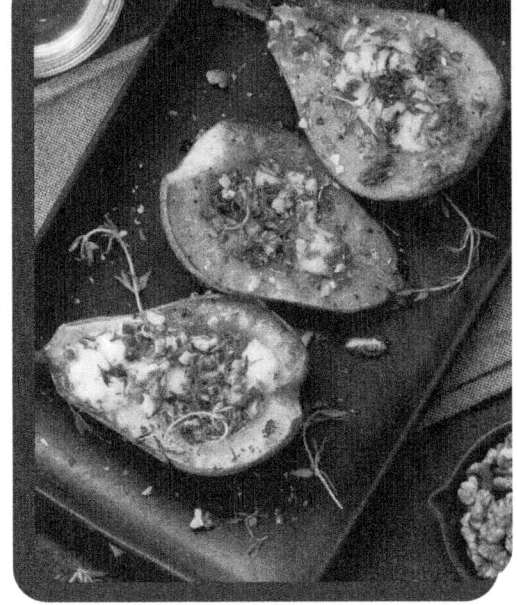

DIRECTIONS

1. Preheat oven to 180C.
2. Cut pears in half, leaving the stems intact.
3. Scoop out the core with a spoon and place pears on a baking tray cut-side up.
4. Sprinkle brown sugar over the pears and cover with foil. Bake for 30 minutes or until soft but still holding their shape.
5. Add Roquefort, honey, walnuts, thyme, and chilli flakes to a small bowl and mix to combine. Fill the pears with the filling and return to the oven to cook, uncovered for 8 – 10 minutes, or until the cheese has melted and the filling is hot.

Individual Platters

SERVES 6 - 10

- Assorted crackers, lavosh and crispbread
- ½ rockmelon, skin and seeds removed, cut into wedges
- Sliced prosciutto
- Salami/Sopressa
- Dip
- Brie
- Blue cheese

- 100 g raw honeycomb
- 50 g muscatels
- 300 g grapes
- Fresh figs or cherries
- 80 g sundried tomatoes
- 150 g mixed pitted olives
- 80 g caperberries
- Quince paste

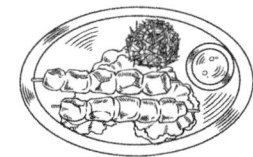

DIRECTIONS

1. Build individual smorgasbord plates, or one large platter, by arranging the ingredients to compliment each other. Wrap rockmelon wedges with prosciutto or pile it proudly on top, adorn brie with raw honeycomb, and pair plump fresh fruit with salty deli delights.
2. Build the plate to be full and generous, and match colours throughout the plate to create contrast and texture.

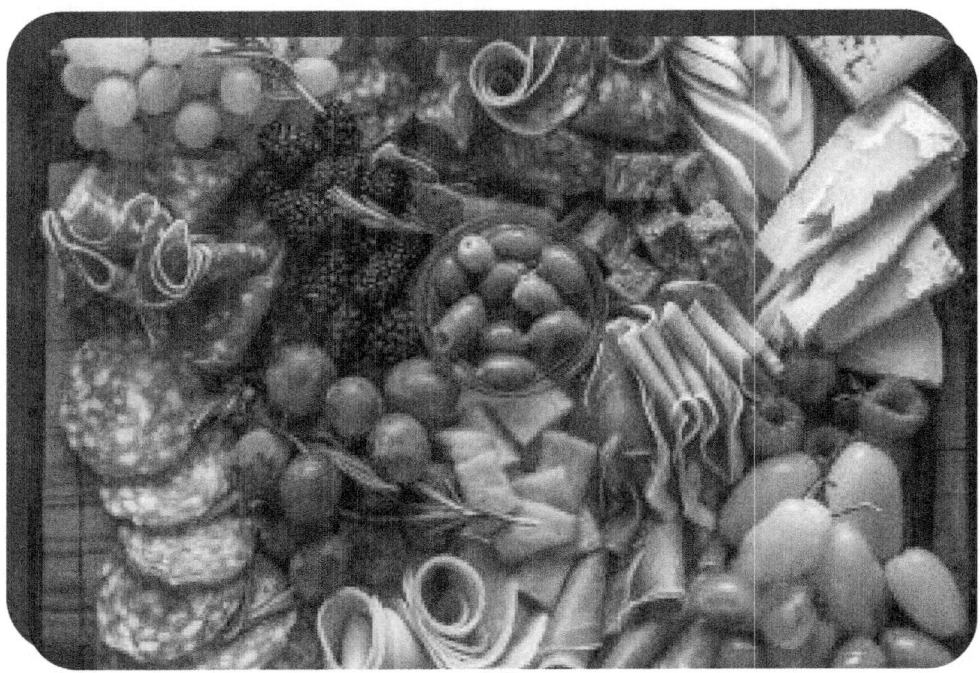

Sumac Labneh

SERVES 6

- 4 beurre bosc pears
- 2 tsp brown sugar
- 80 g Roquefort, crumbled
- 2 tbsp honey
- 10 walnuts, roughly chopped
- 1 tbsp thyme leaves
- 1 tsp chilli flakes, plus extra for garnish

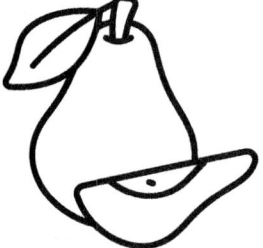

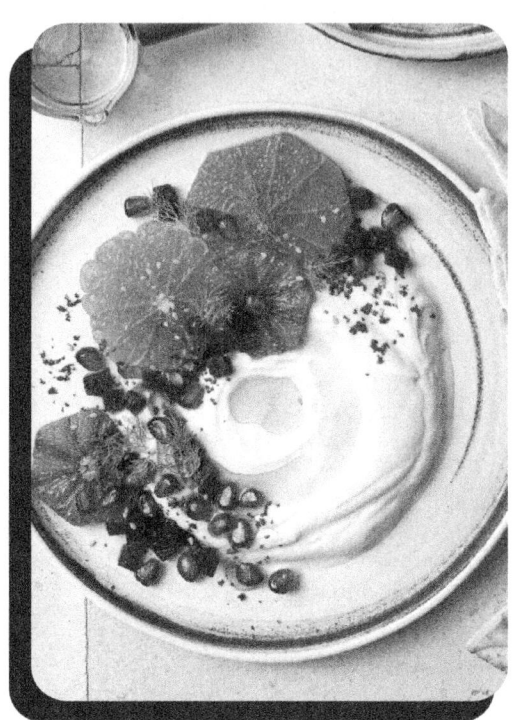

DIRECTIONS

1. Make labneh by lining a sieve with muslin. Add yoghurt and salt to a bowl and mix well. Pour into the muslin, then bring corners of muslin together to form a tight ball. Place the sieve over a bowl to collect liquid and put in the fridge to drain for 24 hours.
2. Dollop labneh onto serving plates. Sprinkle lightly with sumac and drizzle olive oil over labneh. Arrange grapefruit, beetroot, and pomegranate arils on plates and garnish with fennel leaves. Serve with pita bread.

Pizza Pockets

MAKES 40

- 250 g grated mozzarella
- 100 g grated parmesan
- 200 g passata
- 40 g pepperoni, finely diced
- 2 cloves garlic, minced
- 1 tbsp dried basil
- 1 tbsp dried oregano
- 1 tsp dried thyme
- ½ tsp crushed fennel seed
- Pinch chilli flakes
- Pinch of salt
- Pinch of freshly ground black pepper
- 40 square wonton wrappers
- Olive oil for drizzling

DIRECTIONS

1. Preheat oven to 220C. Lightly grease two baking trays. Set aside.
2. In a bowl combine all ingredients except the wonton wrappers and olive oil.
3. Fill a bowl with water. Brush a wonton wrapper with water to lightly dampen it. Add some of the cheese mixture to the centre of the wrapper and then fold the sides of the wrapper over the filling to enclose it. Press gently to seal. Repeat with remaining wonton wrappers and filling.
4. Arrange pizza pockets on baking trays and lightly drizzle with olive oil. Bake for 10-12 minutes or until golden and toasted.

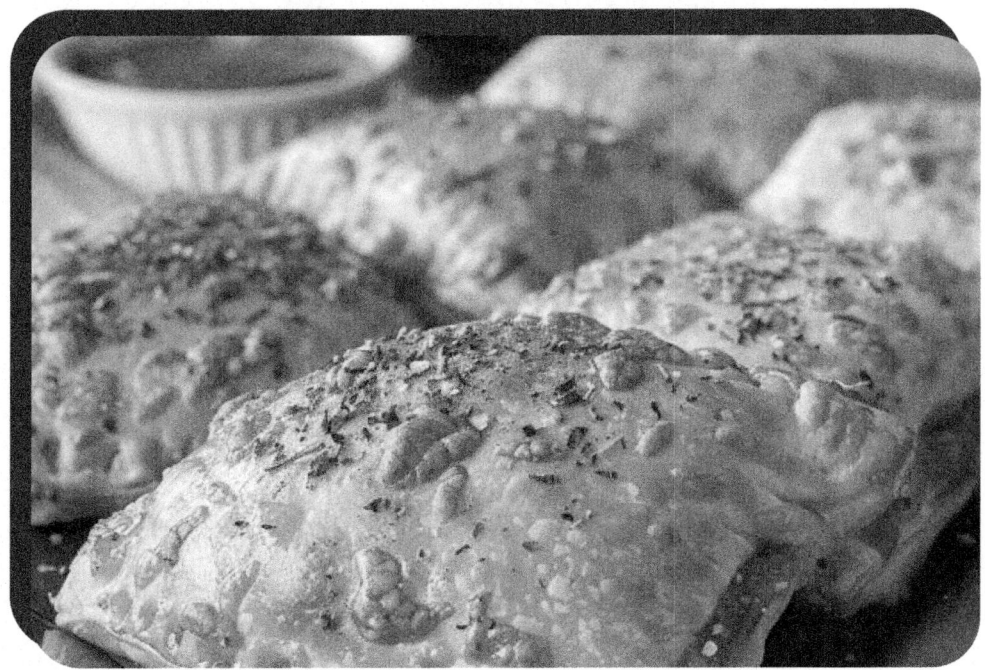

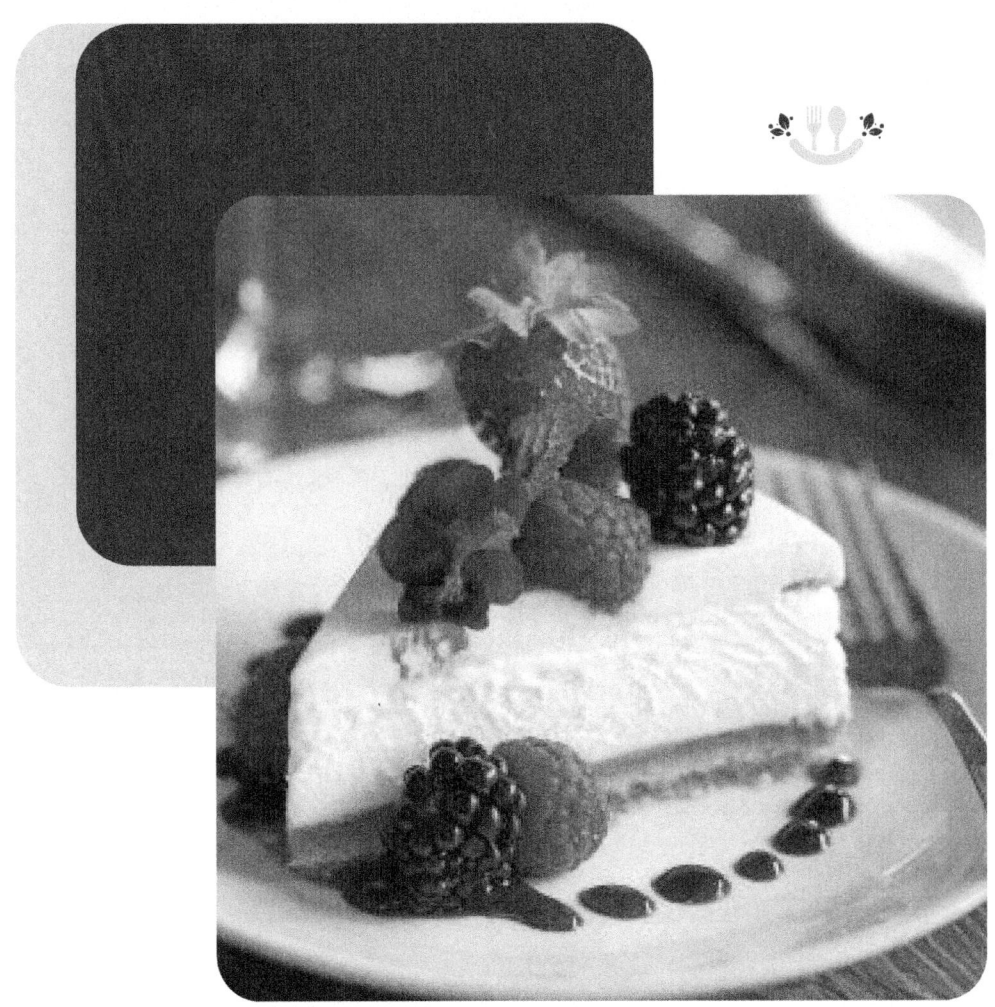

Dessert

"Dessert" is a dish usually served at the end of the main meal to end a meal. Dessert usually has a sweet flavor and can include a variety of foods such as cakes, ice cream, fruit, candy, and many other dishes. The purpose of dessert is not only to provide a delicious taste after a meal but also to create an opportunity for people to sit together, enjoy and chat after the meal.

Very Berry Cheesecake

SERVES 12

- 270g sponge finger biscuits
- 4 ½ cups berries of your choice, divided into 2 equal portions
- 2 cups plus 2 tablespoons of sugar, divided
- 225g cream cheese, softened
- 2 cups whipping cream

DIRECTIONS

1. Combine half the berries and 2 tablespoons of sugar in a bowl. Cover and refrigerate for at least one hour. Meanwhile arrange sponge finger biscuits in the bottom and around the edge of a spring-form pan and set aside.
2. Mix cream cheese in a large mixing bowl until smooth. Gradually beat in the remaining sugar. In a separate bowl whip the cream until stiff peaks form and then fold the cream into the cream cheese.
3. Spoon half the combined mixture over the top of the sponge finger biscuit base. Spread with half the berry and sugar mixture leaving 2.5cm around the edge clear. Then add another layer of sponge finger biscuits over the top and cover with cream cheese mixture. Cover and refrigerate overnight. When ready to serve, remove the sides of the pan and top with reserved berries.

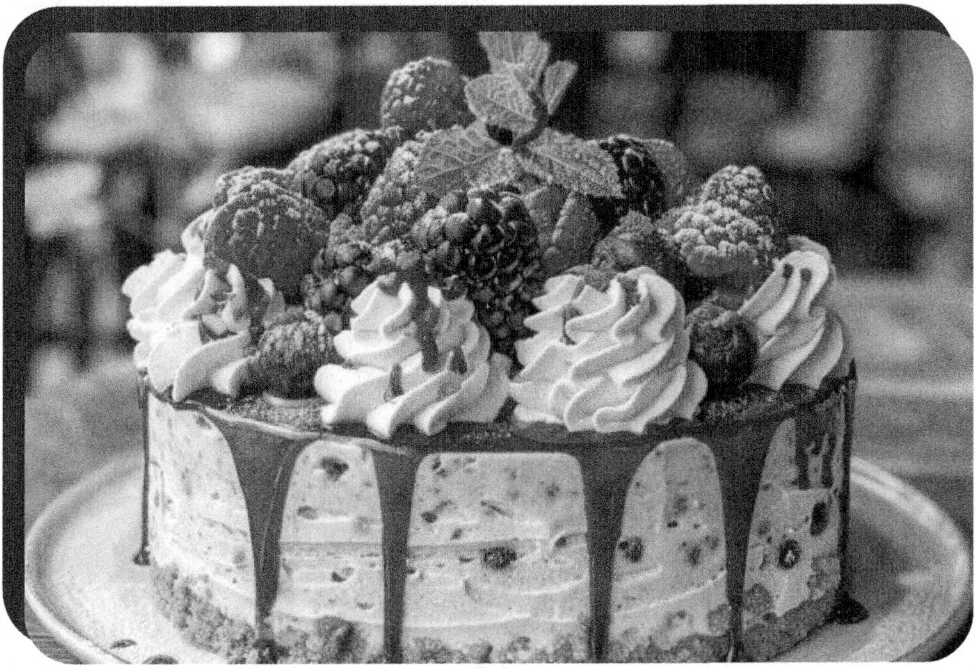

Poached pear with chocolate sauce

SERVES 4

- For the pears
- 75g golden caster sugar
- 1 stick of cinnamon
- 2 strips lemon zest (use a potato peeler)
- 1 star anise
- 1 vanilla pod, split lengthways
- 5 cloves
- 1 piece of fresh root ginger, peeled and sliced
- 4 ripe pears, peeled
- For the chocolate sauce
- 200g good-quality dark chocolate
- 142ml (or ½ cup and 1 tbsp) double cream
- 150ml full-fat milk
- Pinch ground cinnamon
- Valhalla vanilla ice cream, to serve

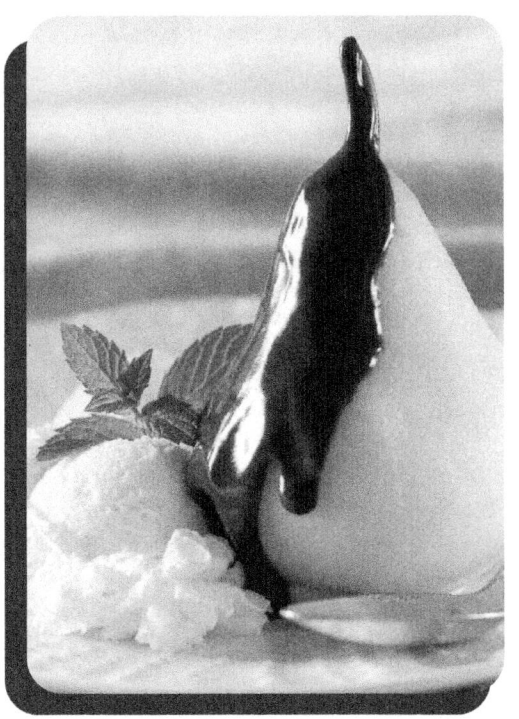

DIRECTIONS

1. In a pot big enough to hold the pears snugly, tip in all the caster sugar, cinnamon, lemon zest, star anise, vanilla, cloves and ginger. Half fill the pot with water and bring to the boil.
2. Simmer for 10 minutes to infuse, then drop in pears, cover and gently poach for about 30 minutes until soft. Turn off the heat and set aside. The pears can be poached up to 2 days ahead and kept in the poaching syrup in the fridge.
3. To make the chocolate sauce, place the chocolate into a heatproof bowl. In a pot, bring the cream, milk and cinnamon to the boil and pour over the chocolate. Stir until the chocolate has melted.
4. To serve, drain the pears and, holding them by the stem, dip them in the chocolate sauce to completely cover. Serve each pear with a generous scoop of vanilla ice cream.

Chocolate Truffles

MAKES 25

- 300 ml double cream
- 300 g good quality dark chocolate, chopped (minimum 65% cocoa solids)
- 1 tsp salt
- Cocoa powder*

DIRECTIONS

1. Place the cream in a pan over a medium heat and bring up to a simmer.
2. Melt the chocolate in a large bowl over a saucepan of simmering water.
3. When the cream is simmering, remove the pan from the heat, add the salt, and add to the melted chocolate in three batches, making sure that the cream is thoroughly incorporated after each addition.
4. Pour the chocolate mixture into a bowl and leave to cool at room temperature for 2 hours, then place in the fridge for 5-6 hours or until set.
5. Using a small melon baller, scoop balls of the chocolate out of the ganache then roll in cocoa powder before serving.

* Add a splash of your favourite liqueur to the ganache, we like Baileys but you can add anything that you like. Try different coatings for the truffles like white, milk or dark chocolate or add a few drops of food colouring to sugar or coconut before coating truffles.

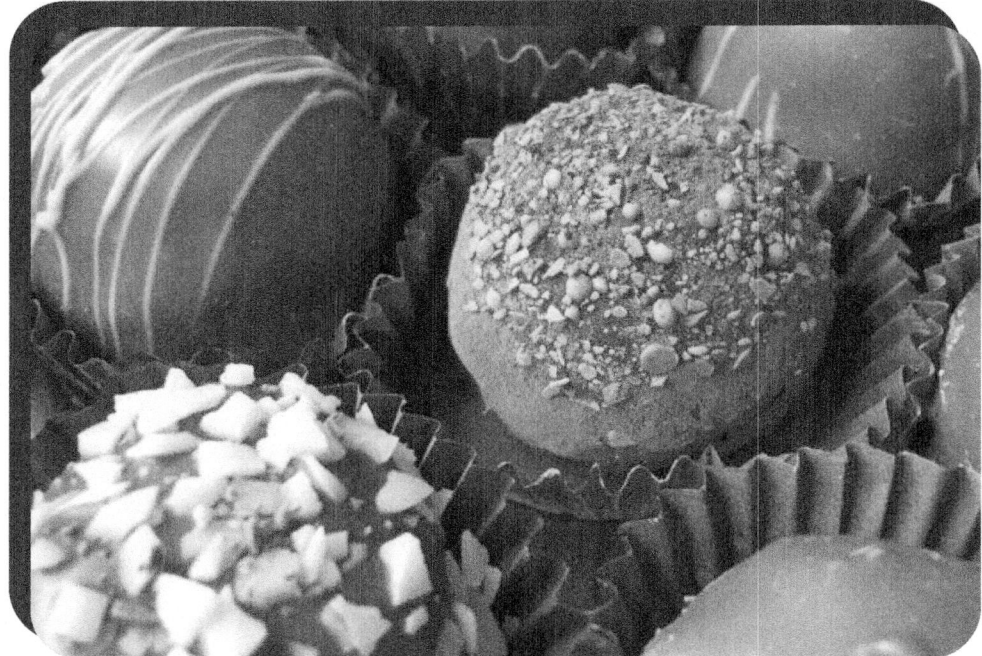

Homemade waffles with Valhalla Ice Cream

MAKES 20

- 200g (1⅓ cups) plain flour
- 2 tablespoons olive oil
- 2 teaspoons sweet sherry
- 2 tablespoons caster sugar
- 3 eggs, separated
- 1 cup milk
- For greasing: soft butter
- Island Berries Chocolate Sauce
- Valhalla Vanilla Bean Ice Cream

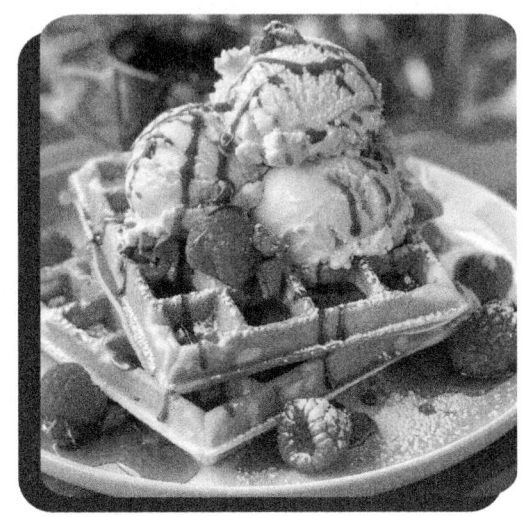

DIRECTIONS

1. For waffles, sift flour into a bowl with a pinch of salt, add oil, sherry, sugar and egg yolks, then stir to combine.
2. Gradually add milk, whisking continuously, until a smooth batter forms.
3. Using an electric mixer, whisk egg whites until soft peaks form.
4. Fold egg whites into waffle batter.
5. Heat a greased waffle iron on medium heat then cook ⅓ cup of waffle batter at a time for 2 minutes, then turn waffle iron over and cook for another 2 minutes or until waffle is crisp and golden.
6. Serve waffles immediately, topped with your favourite Valhalla ice cream and drizzled with Island Berries Chocolate Sauce.

Molten chocolate lava cakes

SERVES 8

- 200g dark chocolate, chopped
- 200g butter, chopped
- 200g caster sugar
- 200g plain flour, sifted
- 4 eggs plus 4 extra egg yolks
- Extra butter for greasing
- Cocoa powder for dusting

DIRECTIONS

1. Grease 8 small ramekins with the extra butter.
2. Line the base of each ramekin with a circle of baking paper.
3. Sprinkle a little cocoa powder into the base of each ramekin and shake it until the sides are covered. Shake off any excess cocoa powder and set ramekins aside.
4. Heat butter and chocolate in microwave at 50% power for 3-4 minutes, stirring every 30 seconds until melted and smooth. Set aside to cool at room temperature.
5. Using electric blender whisk eggs plus extra yolks and caster sugar in a bowl until pale and smooth.
6. Add ¼ of egg mix to chocolate and beat until smooth. Repeat with remaining egg mixture until it is all added to chocolate.
7. Fold in flour.
8. Divide mixture between the ramekins and refrigerate for 1 hour.
9. Preheat oven to 180C.
10. Put ramekins on a baking tray and place in oven.
11. Cook for 10-12 minutes or until cakes are beginning to come away from the sides of the ramekins.
12. Remove from oven and allow to rest for 2 minutes.
13. Loosen cakes from the sides of the ramekins and upturn onto a plate.
14. Remove baking paper and dust with cocoa powder or icing sugar to serve.
15. Enjoy with cream or ice-cream.

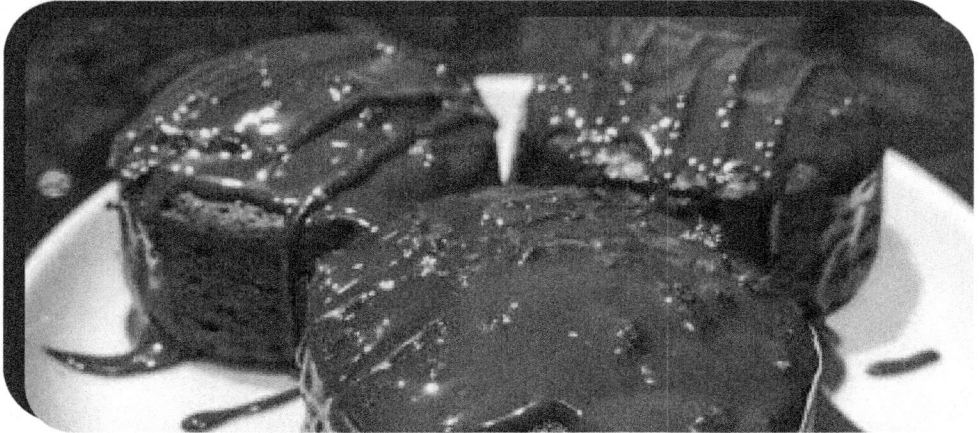

Coconut cream, white chocolate and kiwi fruit tartlets

MAKES 8 TARTLETS

- 240g Gingernut or Butternut Snap biscuits
- 200g unsalted butter
- 125ml coconut milk
- 250g white chocolate, chopped
- Kiwi fruit, thinly sliced, to serve
- Dessicated coconut, to serve

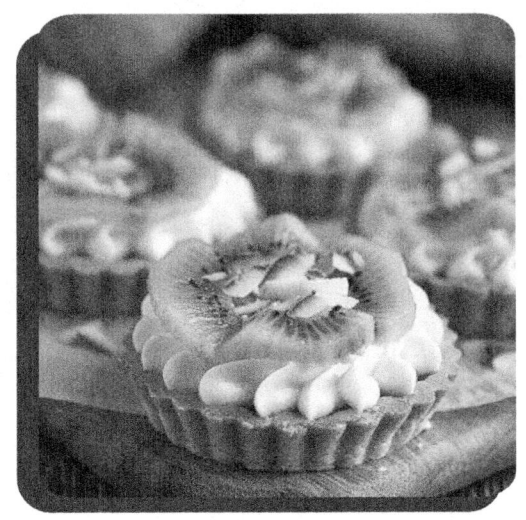

DIRECTIONS

1. Grease eight 10cm loose-bottomed tart pans.
2. Blend biscuits in a food processor until the texture is a fine crumb.
3. Melt 100g of the butter, then add to the biscuits and process to combine. Press into the base and sides of the tart pans.
4. Put the remaining 100g butter with the coconut milk in a saucepan and bring to the boil, then remove from the heat.
5. Add white chocolate and stir until smooth. Pour into tart shells and chill for 2 hours or until set.
6. Serve topped with kiwi fruit slices and shaved coconut.

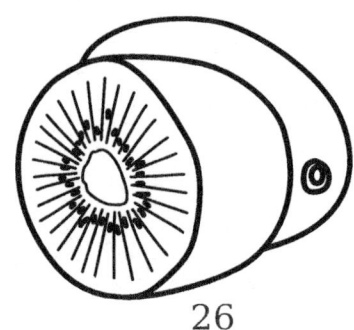

Chocolate coated cheesecake balls

MAKES APPROXIMATELY 20
- 225g cream cheese, softened
- 4 tbsp butter, softened
- ½ cup plain sweet biscuits
- 4 cups icing sugar
- 285g milk cooking chocolate
- 50g hazelnuts, finely chopped

DIRECTIONS
1. Use a food processor to blitz the biscuits into a fine crumb.
2. In a large bowl, combine cream cheese and butter. Fold in the biscuit crumbs and mix well.
3. Add icing sugar, one cup at a time and mix well. Cover and put in the fridge for 2 hours.
4. Use an ice-cream scoop or two spoons to scoop out batter into balls and place them on a tray lined with baking paper. Return to the fridge for a further 10 minutes.
5. While balls are in the fridge, melt the chocolate in the microwave or over a double-boiler on the stovetop.
6. Place a ball on a fork and dip in the chocolate, making sure to coat it fully and then sprinkle with hazelnuts. Repeat for remaining balls.
7. Refrigerate balls until ready to serve.

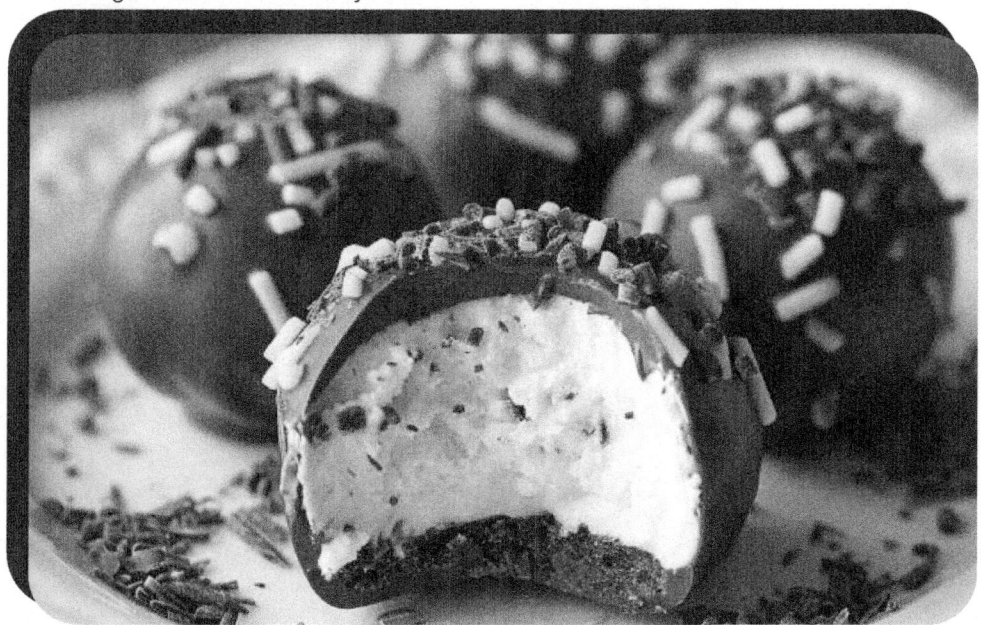

Kiwi, mint and lime ice-cream pops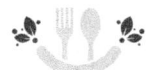

SERVES 6

- Icy pole moulds
- 2 cups fruit juice – we blended kiwi fruit, a handful of mint leaves and the juice of 1 lime to create the vibrant green colour and delicious flavour of our ice-cream pops
- 500ml vanilla ice-cream, softened

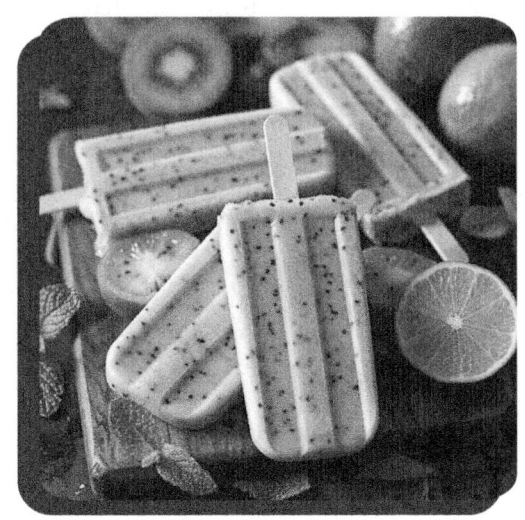

DIRECTIONS

1. Divide softened ice-cream evenly between the icy-pole moulds and insert sticks. Freeze for 4 hours until very hard.
2. Blitz peeled kiwi fruit, mint leaves and the juice of 1 lime until juiced.
3. Remove ice-cream from moulds and set aside.
4. Pour juice into the moulds, dividing evenly. Only fill about 1/3 of the mould with juice as it will displace when the ice-cream is returned to the mould.
5. Gently put the ice-cream back into the mould and return to the freezer. Leave to set overnight before unmoulding and enjoying.

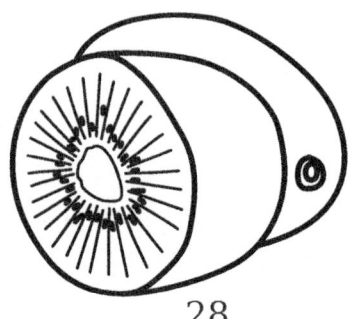

Kiwi, coconut and watermelon pops

MAKES 10
- 3 ½ cups cubed seedless watermelon
- 4 tablespoons sugar, divided (optional)
- ¾ tablespoon lemon juice
- ½ cup canned coconut milk, well shaken
- 6 medium kiwi fruit
- Icy- pole molds

DIRECTIONS
1. The sugar in this recipe is optional and can be omitted depending on your preference.
2. Add watermelon, 1 ½ tablespoons sugar and lemon juice to a blender and blend to a puree.
3. Skim off foam and carefully pour into 10 icy-pole molds, filling to about 2/3 full.
4. Cover with the lid and insert the icy-pole sticks and freeze for three hours. You will need to give them a stir every 30 minutes as the watermelon juice tends to separate.
5. After three hours, whisk coconut milk with 1 tablespoon of sugar until dissolved and chill for 30 minutes. The consistency should be pouring consistency and not too thick. If it has thickened too much add a couple of tablespoons of water to thin it out.
6. Remove the popsicles from the freezer and pour 1 tablespoon of coconut milk mix in an even layer over the watermelon layer. Return to freezer and chill uncovered for 45 minutes.
7. Peel the kiwi fruit and transfer the fruit to a blender with the remaining sugar. Pulse until pureed. Rub through a fine mesh strainer to remove seeds and then chill the puree for 30 minutes.
8. Take the popsicles from the freezer and top each with about a tablespoon of the kiwifruit mix. Return to the freezer and chill until popsicles are fully set, about 2 - 3 hours.
9. When ready to eat, carefully remove the pops from their molds and enjoy!

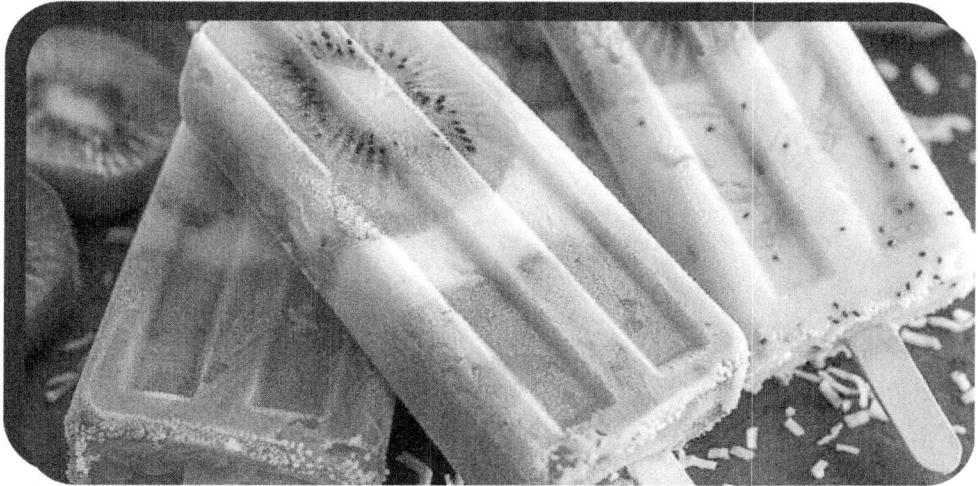

Pina Colada Nice Cream

SERVES 4

- 4 x 400ml cans of coconut cream, plus coconut water
- 3 cups freshly chopped pineapple, plus extra for garnish
- 1/4 cup Malibu rum
- Toasted sweetened coconut, for garnish

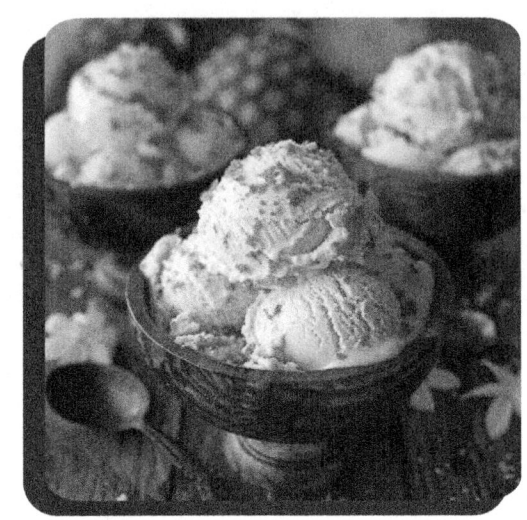

DIRECTIONS

1. Turn over cans of coconut cream and chill in the fridge at least 3 hours, ideally overnight. When ready to whip, turn right-side-up and open.
2. Spoon coconut cream into a large bowl and use a hand mixer to beat until creamy. Set aside.
3. In a blender, blend pineapple with rum and the reserved coconut water from one can.
4. Fold pineapple mixture into whipped coconut cream until combined, then transfer to a 22 x 12cm baking dish.
5. Garnish with more pineapple and toasted coconut.
6. Freeze until firm, approximately 4 hours, then serve.

Chocolate and zucchini loaf cake

MAKES 8

- 1/2 cup caster sugar
- 1/2 cup firmly packed brown sugar
- 1/2 cup vegetable oil
- 1 tsp vanilla extract
- 2 eggs
- Pinch salt
- 1/2 tsp cinnamon
- 1/2 cup cocoa powder
- 1 cup plain flour
- 1/2 tsp baking powder
- 1 tsp baking soda
- 1 1/2 cups firmly packed grated zucchini (about 4 small zucchini)

DIRECTIONS

1. Preheat oven to 180°C. Grease and line a loaf tin with baking paper.
2. Place the sugars, oil, vanilla, eggs, salt and cinnamon in a mixing bowl.
3. Whisk together until combined. Sift in the cocoa powder, flour, baking powder and baking soda.
4. Using a rubber spatula, fold the dry mixture into the wet mixture until just combined. Add the grated zucchini and stir through.
5. Pour the mixture into the prepared loaf tin and bake for 50-60 minutes, or until a skewer inserted into the centre comes out clean.

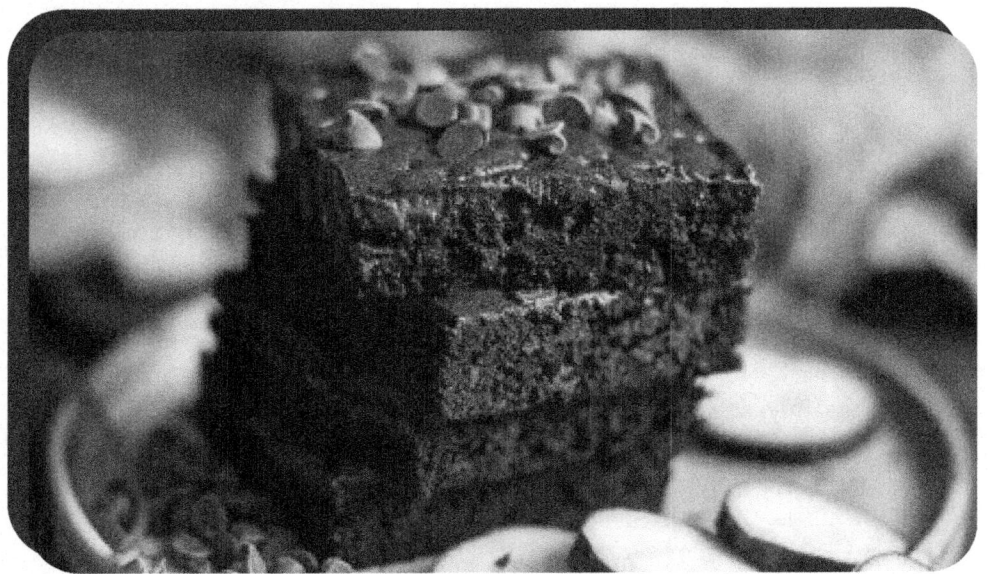

Coconut slice with lemon curd

MAKES 16

- 80g unsalted butter
- 200g Arnott's Marie biscuits
- 2 cups desiccated coconut
- 1/3 cup honey
- ¾ cup coconut oil

For the lemon curd

- 4 lemons
- ½ cup caster sugar
- 1 egg
- 3 egg yolks
- 3 tbsp cornflour

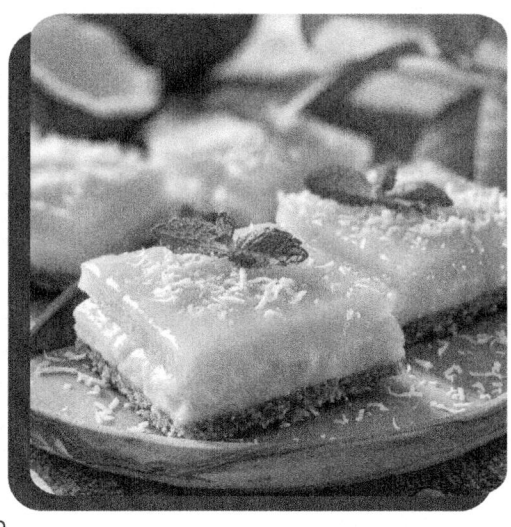

DIRECTIONS

1. Melt butter in a small saucepan.
2. Crush biscuits with a food processor until they are fine and crumbly.
3. Add melted butter to biscuits and continue processing until they are the consistency of wet sand.
4. Press the biscuit mixture into base of a 20cm cake pan lined with baking paper. Ensure base is evenly covered. Place in freezer while you make the filling.
5. Next make coconut filling.
6. The coconut oil needs to be the consistency of soft butter. If yours is too firm, you can warm it gently in a small saucepan until just melted. Add honey and coconut to coconut oil and stir to combine.
7. Remove base from the freezer and top with coconut filling. Smooth and press down the top with the back of a spoon. Place the pan back in the freezer while you prepare the lemon curd topping.
8. Juice the lemons.
9. In a large mixing bowl, whisk together the lemon juice, sugar, eggs and cornflour.
10. Pour mixture into a medium saucepan and cook over medium heat until it thickens. Set aside to cool slightly.
11. Pour the lemon curd over the slice and place in the fridge to cool completely, about 1 hour.
12. When the lemon curd has cooled and set, remove from fridge and slice using a sharp knife. You will find it easier to slice if you heat the knife under hot water first. Cut into 5cm x 5cm pieces. These will keep, refrigerated for 4-5 days.

Berry Ice Cream Popsicles

MAKES 6-8 POPSICLES
- 2 cups blueberries (or berries of your choice)
- 2 tbsp honey
- 2 cups vanilla yoghurt

DIRECTIONS

1. Blitz blueberries in a food processor on high speed until they are partially liquified but still have some chunks.
2. Add honey and stir well to combine.
3. Add yoghurt and gently mix. Taste mix and add extra honey if you would like the popsicles to be sweeter.
4. Pour mixture into popsicle moulds. Freeze for 2 hours, then put a wooden popsicle stick in the middle. Return to freezer and freeze overnight.
5. When ready to serve run popsicle moulds under warm water to make them easy to remove.

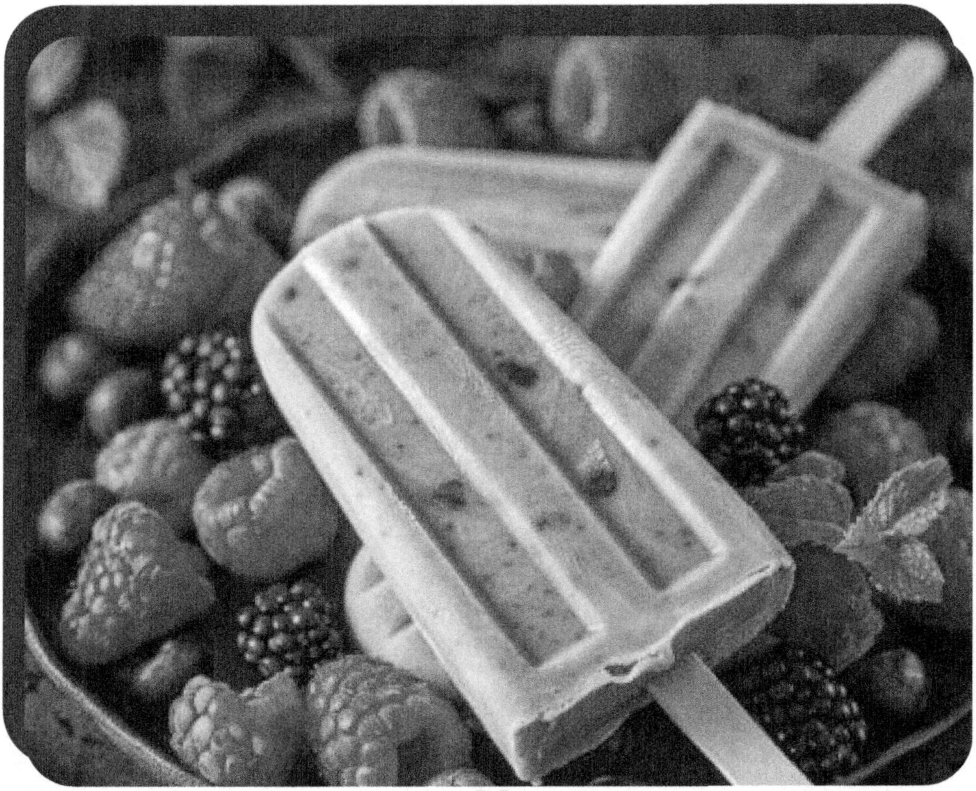

Raspberry and Pistachio Semifreddo

SERVES 8

- 2 eggs
- 4 egg yolks
- 1/3 cup caster sugar
- 1 3/4 cups thickened cream, whipped
- 1 cup pistachio nut kernels, roasted, roughly chopped
- 1 tablespoon rosewater
- Mint leaves to serve
- 200g fresh raspberries plus additional 100g fresh raspberries to serve

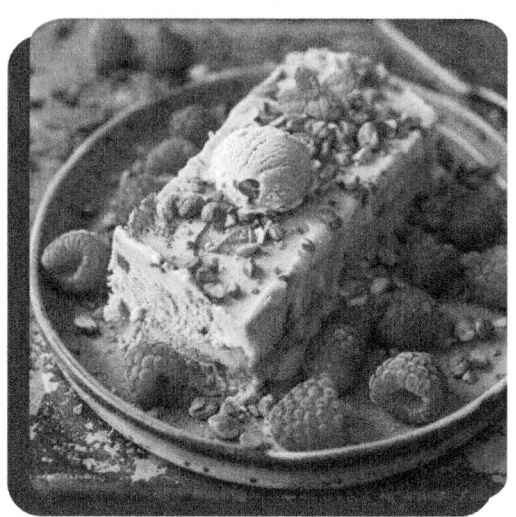

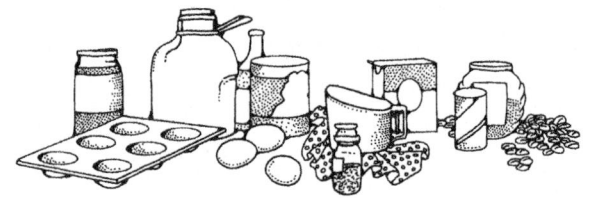

DIRECTIONS

1. Grease a 19cm long x 6cm deep loaf pan. Line with baking paper and leave a 5cm overhang on both ends.
2. Bring a saucepan of water to a simmer. In a heatproof bowl place eggs, egg yolks and sugar. Place bowl over a saucepan and whisk ingredients for 4 to 5 minutes or until thick and creamy.
3. Remove from heat and whisk for a further 5 minutes or until cool.
4. Transfer the mixture to a large bowl and fold in cream, 2/3 cup pistachios, 200g raspberries and rosewater.
5. Pour mixture into prepared loaf pan.
6. Cover and place in freezer overnight.
7. Stand at room temperature for 5 minutes before turning out on a plate. Top with remaining raspberries and pistachios and mint leaves to serve.

Orange and Lemon Poppy Seed Cake

SERVES 6

- 1/3 cup poppy seeds
- ¼ cup milk
- 125 g butter, softened
- 1 cup caster sugar
- 3 eggs
- 2 tbsp grated orange rind, divided
- 2 tsp grated lemon rind, divided
- 2 cups self-raising flour
- ½ cup sour cream
- ¼ cup orange juice

For the Icing
- ½ cup icing sugar
- 2 tbsp lemon juice

DIRECTIONS

1. Preheat oven to 160C. Grease and line a loaf tin.
2. Pour poppy seeds into a small bowl and add milk. Stir and set aside to soak.
3. Beat butter and sugar until pale and creamy. Add eggs one at a time, beating well between each addition. Add half of the orange rind and half the lemon rind and stir to incorporate.
4. Sift in flour, then add sour cream, orange juice and the poppy seeds and milk. Mix gently to combine.
5. Put batter into prepared loaf tin and bake for 40-45 minutes or until a skewer inserted comes out clean.
6. Cook in tin for 15 minutes before turning out to cool on a wire rack.
7. To make the icing, combine lemon juice and icing sugar and stir with a fork until smooth. If more liquid is required add water or extra lemon juice.
8. Spread icing over cake and garnish with remaining orange and lemon rind.

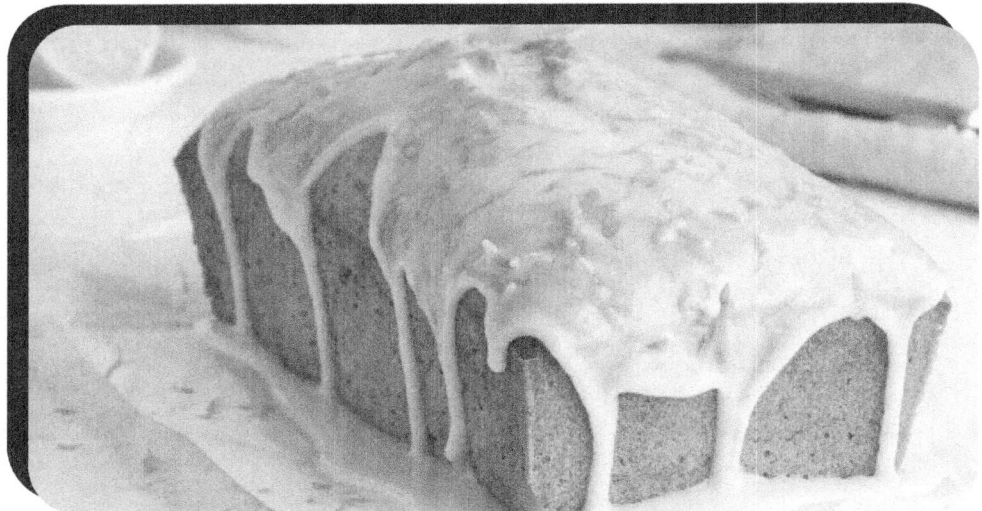

Choc Orange Biscuits

MAKES 15

For the chocolate orange cream
- 200ml cream
- 200g milk chocolate, roughly chopped
- 1 orange, zested

For the biscuits
- 200g unsalted butter, softened
- 200g brown sugar
- 125g caster sugar
- 2 eggs, lightly beaten
- 1 tsp vanilla extract
- 400g plain flour, sifted
- 1 tsp bicarbonate of soda
- 1 tsp baking powder
- Pinch of salt
- 200g dark chocolate, chopped

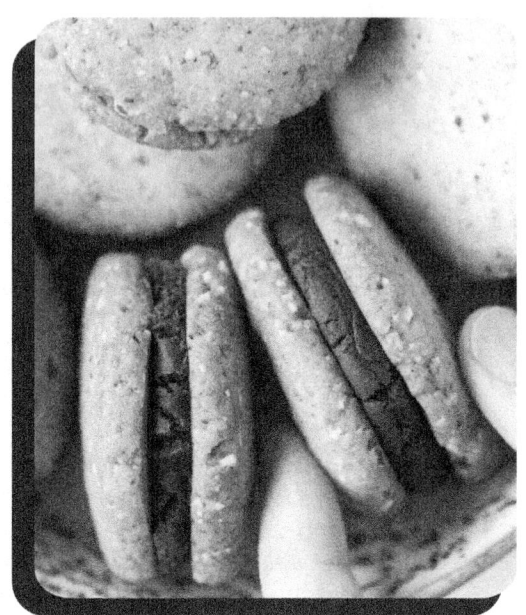

DIRECTIONS
1. Preheat oven to 190C.
2. Place cream in a small saucepan and bring to the boil. Reduce heat to low and add chocolate and stir until it has melted and the mixture is shiny. Remove from the heat and stir through the orange zest. Pour into a bowl and refrigerate until the cream is set (approximately 2 hours). The consistency should be set but still spreadable.
3. Using an electric blender beat butter and sugar until light and fluffy. Add eggs gradually, whisking as they are added. Add vanilla and blend to combine. Add flour, bicarb, baking powder and salt and mix until the mixture comes together into a dough.
4. Add chopped chocolate, folding it well to incorporate the chocolate pieces through the biscuit dough.
5. Use a teaspoon to scoop out pieces of the dough and roll them into balls. Place balls on lined baking trays, leaving plenty of room for the biscuits to spread during cooking. Bake in batches for 10 -15 minutes or until golden. Remove from oven and set aside to cool.
6. When the biscuits have completely cooled, spread half the batch with the chocolate orange cream and sandwich together with the remaining biscuits.

Watermelon, Feta and Mint Appetiser

SERVES 6

- ¼ to ½ a watermelon
- 125g feta cheese
- Balsamic vinegar for drizzling
- Fresh mint leaves to garnish

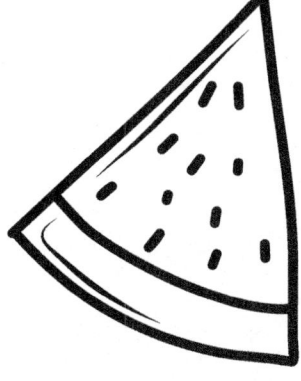

DIRECTIONS

1. Cut watermelon into six 5cm x 5cm squares
2. Crumble over feta, garnish with mint leaves and drizzle with balsamic vinegar.

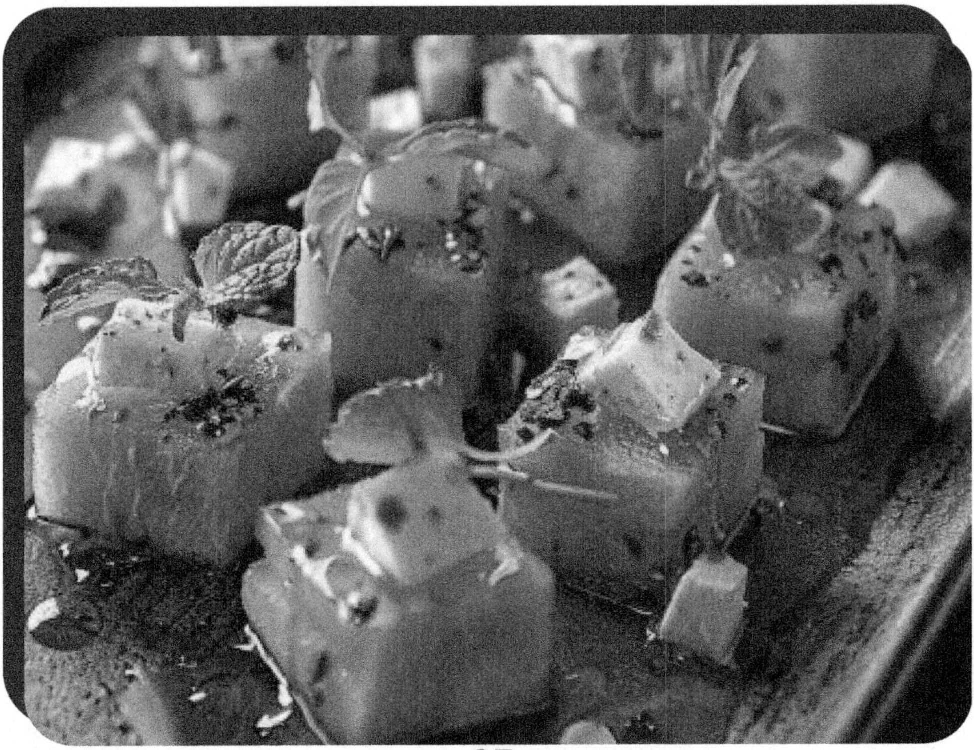

Traditional Anzac Biscuits

MAKES 35

- 2 cups rolled oats
- 1 cup plain flour
- 2/3 cup caster sugar
- 2/3 cup desiccated coconut
- ¾ cup golden syrup
- 125g unsalted butter
- 1 teaspoon bicarbonate of soda
- 2 tablespoons hot water

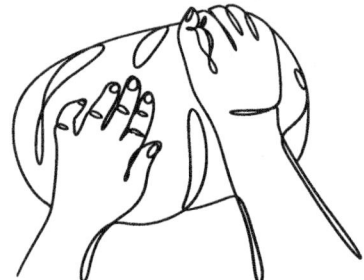

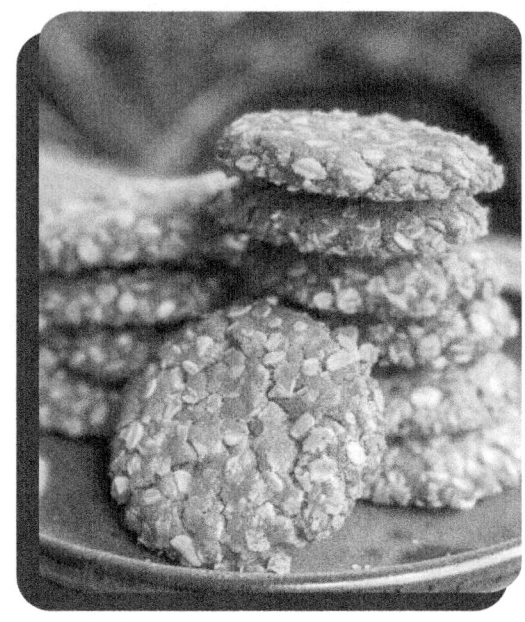

DIRECTIONS

1. Preheat oven to 160°C. Place the oats, flour, sugar and coconut in a bowl and mix to combine.
2. Place the golden syrup and butter in a saucepan over low heat and cook, stirring, until melted. Combine the bicarbonate of soda with the water and add to the butter mixture. Pour into the oat mixture and mix well to combine.
3. Place tablespoonfuls of the mixture onto baking trays lined with non-stick baking paper and flatten to 7cm rounds, allowing room to spread. Bake for 8-10 minutes or until deep golden. Allow to cool on baking trays for 5 minutes before transferring to wire racks to cool completely.

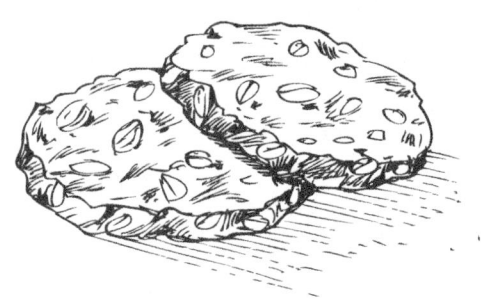

Brie Stuffed Pretzels with Rosemary and Sea Salt

MAKES 8 PRETZELS

- 1½ cup warm water
- 1 Tbsp sugar
- 2 tsp sea salt
- 2¼ tsp instant yeast
- 4½ cups plain flour
- 60g butter, melted
- 220g Mon Pere brie, sliced
- 8 cups water
- ½ cup baking soda
- Olive oil, for brushing
- Sea salt
- Fresh rosemary, for garnish

DIRECTIONS

1. In the bowl of an electric mixer, mix together water, sugar, salt and yeast; let sit for 5 minutes until frothy.
2. Using the dough hook, add the flour and butter, mixing on low speed until dough pulls away from the sides of the bowl, approximately 5 minutes.
3. Transfer dough to a lightly oiled bowl, cover with plastic wrap and set aside in a warm place for about an hour or until the dough has doubled in size.
4. Turn the dough out onto a lightly floured surface and divide into 8 equal pieces.
5. Roll each piece into a 45 centimetre rope, then flatten rope so it's more of a long rectangle. Place brie cheese in the centre, then roll dough back into a rope shape, pinching the edges to ensure all the cheese is completely encased in the dough. Shape into pretzels.
6. When ready to eat, preheat the oven to 220°C. Line two large baking trays with baking paper; set aside.
7. Bring the water and baking soda to a boil in a large saucepan.
8. Using a flat spatula, drop the pretzels into the boiling water and boil for 30 seconds. Depending on the size of your saucepan you may need to boil one at a time.
9. Remove pretzels from the water, drain and place on the baking sheets. Brush the top of each pretzel with olive oil, sprinkle with sea salt and fresh rosemary.
10. Bake until golden and puffed, 12-14 minutes. Serve warm.

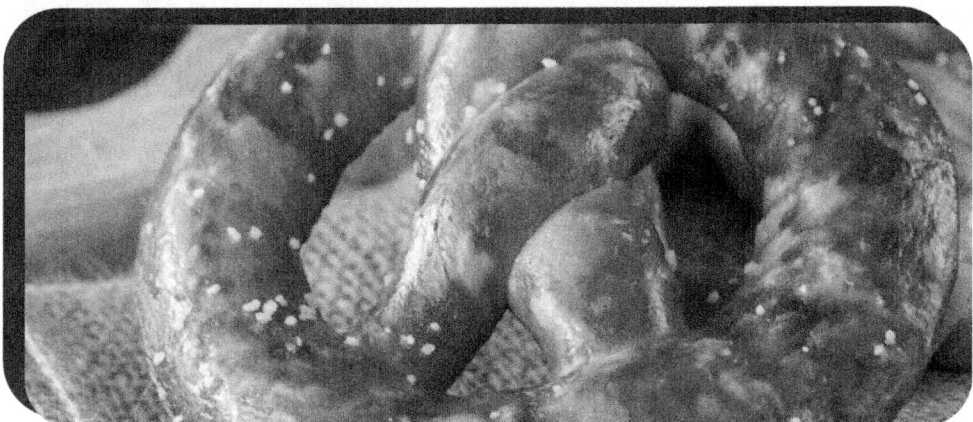

Gluten Free Christmas Fruit Mince Pies

MAKES APPROXIMATELY 12

- 225 g plain gluten free flour
- ½ tsp xanthan gum
- 100 g unsalted butter, chilled and cut into cubes
- 70 g icing sugar
- 2 large free range eggs
- 350 g fruit mince
- 2 tbsp caster sugar

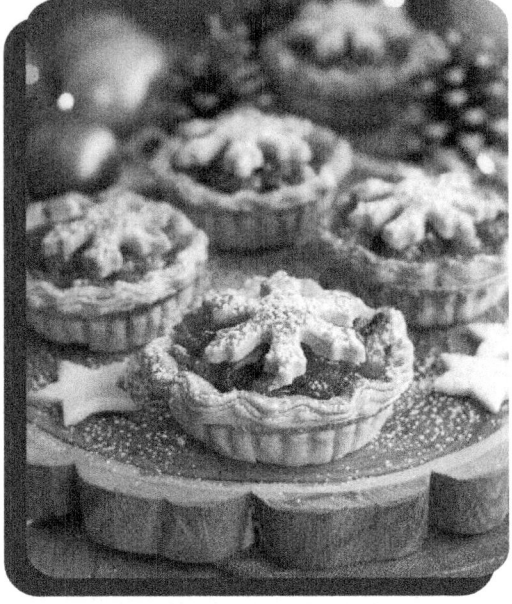

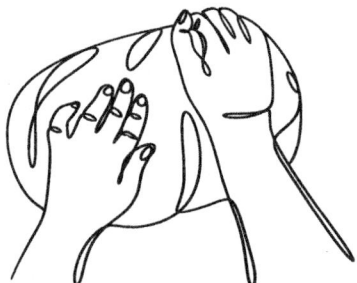

DIRECTIONS

1. Add sifted flour and xanthan gum to a large bowl and stir to combine.
2. Add cubed butter and rub it into the flour with your fingers until it is the texture of breadcrumbs.
3. Add icing sugar and stir to combine, then add 1 egg and mix to form a rough ball.
4. Knead pastry with your hands until it is smooth, then wrap in clingwrap and refrigerate for 1 hour.
5. Preheat oven to 180C and grease a 12 hole regular (not Texas size) muffin tin.
6. Roll pastry out to a 4 millimetre thickness on a lightly floured surface and then use a 7 centimetre cookie cutter to cut out 12 circles. Use a star shaped cookie cutter to cut out 12 stars.
7. Put the pastry circles into the muffin tin, pressing it into the base and sides.
8. Add fruit mince and then top with pastry stars.
9. Whisk remaining egg with a fork and egg wash the stars, then sprinkle with caster sugar and bake for 20-25 minutes or until the pastry is golden brown.
10. Remove from oven and cool.

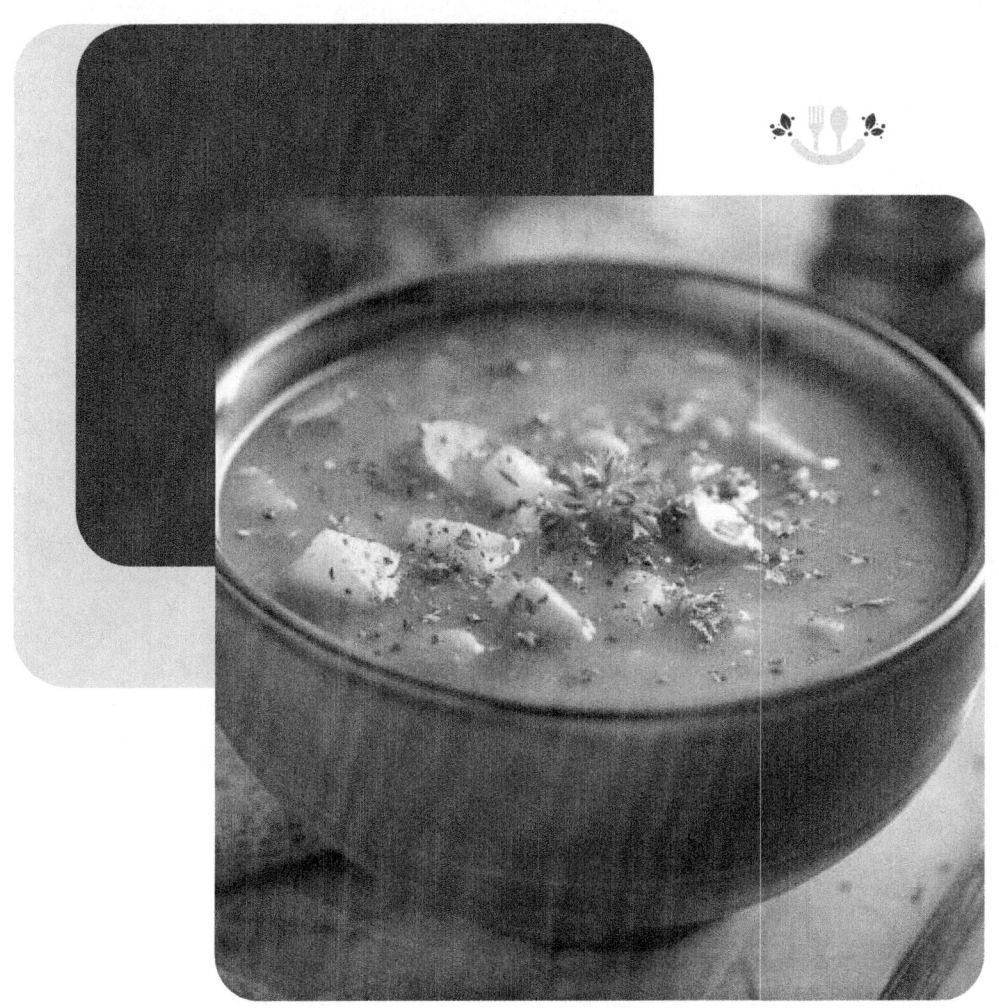

Soup

Soup, also known as soup, is a liquid or semi-liquid dish made from combining water with ingredients such as meat, fish, vegetables, and often spices. Soups can be served hot or cold and are a popular part of meals around the world. Soups provide a source of easily digestible nutrients, often served as an appetizer or as a light main meal. The variety of soups is very rich, depending on local ingredients and culinary traditions of each region.

Hot Soba Noodle Soup with Salmon, Cucumber and Togarashi

SERVES 4

- 2 litres cold water, plus up to ¾ cup additional
- 50g dried kombu or other dried kelp
- 50g bonito flakes
- 2 tsp sea salt
- 1 tbsp sugar
- 4-6 tbsp soy sauce
- 2 tbsp mirin
- 500g dried soba noodles
- 4 spring onions, thinly sliced, white and light green parts only
- 1 bunch watercress, trimmed
- ½ cucumber, thinly sliced
- 4 tbsp grated daikon
- 400g salmon, cut into bite-sized pieces
- Togarashi to garnish

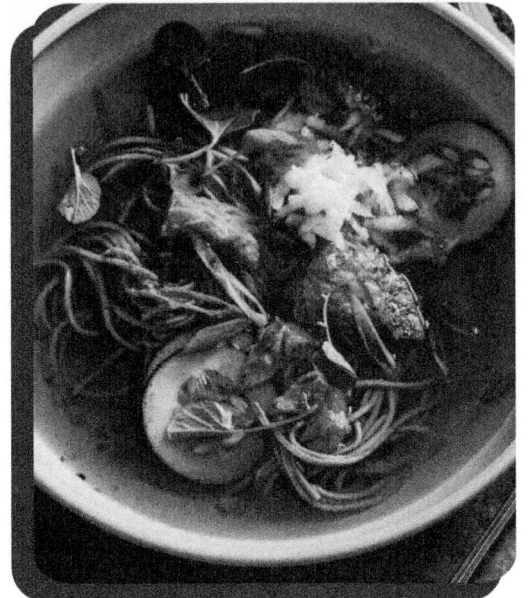

DIRECTIONS

1. Begin by making a dashi – rinse kombu under cold water and place it in a medium saucepan with 2 litres of cold water. Heat over medium-high heat until tiny bubbles form at the edges, about 12 to 14 minutes. Don't let the water come to a full boil. Remove kombu from water with tongs. Add ½ cup cold water and bonito flakes. Bring just to a boil, about 2 minutes, then remove from the heat and cover. Set aside for 10 minutes and then strain through a fine mesh sieve or cheesecloth into another pot. Do not press the bonito flakes.
2. To make the noodle broth add dashi, salt, soy sauce, sugar, mirin plus ½ cup additional water to a large pot over medium-high heat and bring to the boil. Remove from heat.
3. To make noodles – boil noodles according to packet directions. Drain and rinse well under cold water. Shake to remove excess water.
4. To cook salmon – line a baking tray with baking paper and cook in a preheated 180C oven for 5 minutes. Remove and set aside.
5. Divide noodles among four bowls. Add salmon and pour over broth. Top each bowl with vegetables, and togarashi.

Thai chicken coconut soup

SERVES 2

- 125g cellophane noodles
- 6 cups chicken stock
- 1-2 red Thai (or jalapeño) peppers, seeded and finely chopped (plus slices for garnish)
- 1 additional red Thai (or jalapeño) pepper slices for garnish
- 3 cloves garlic, chopped
- 1 tablespoon grated ginger
- 2 teaspoons grated lemon zest
- 1 teaspoon grated lime zest
- 1/4 cup fresh lemon (or lime) juice
- 4 tablespoons Thai fish sauce, divided
- 225g shiitake mushrooms, sliced (3 cups)
- 2 boneless, skinless chicken breasts (about 150g each), cut into 1cm-wide strips
- 1 cup light coconut milk
- 2 cups baby spinach
- 2 tablespoon chopped coriander (plus sprigs for garnish)
- Coriander sprigs for garnish

DIRECTIONS

1. Place noodles in a bowl; add enough warm water to cover and let sit until soft, this will take about 15 minutes.
2. Once soft, drain the noodles. Combine stock, pepper, garlic, ginger, lemon zest, lime zest, lemon juice and 3 tablespoon fish sauce in a medium saucepan. Season with salt. Bring to a simmer, add noodles and cook 3 minutes more.
3. Using tongs, transfer noodles to a bowl and cover with foil to keep warm. Add mushrooms to stock; season with salt, if desired; simmer 3 minutes more. Add chicken and coconut milk and simmer, stirring, until chicken is just cooked, about 3 minutes.
4. Stir in spinach until it begins to wilt, about 1 minute. Add chopped coriander and season with remaining 1 tablespoon fish sauce.
5. Using tongs, divide noodles among 2 bowls. Ladle soup into bowls and garnish with sprigs of coriander and slices of pepper.

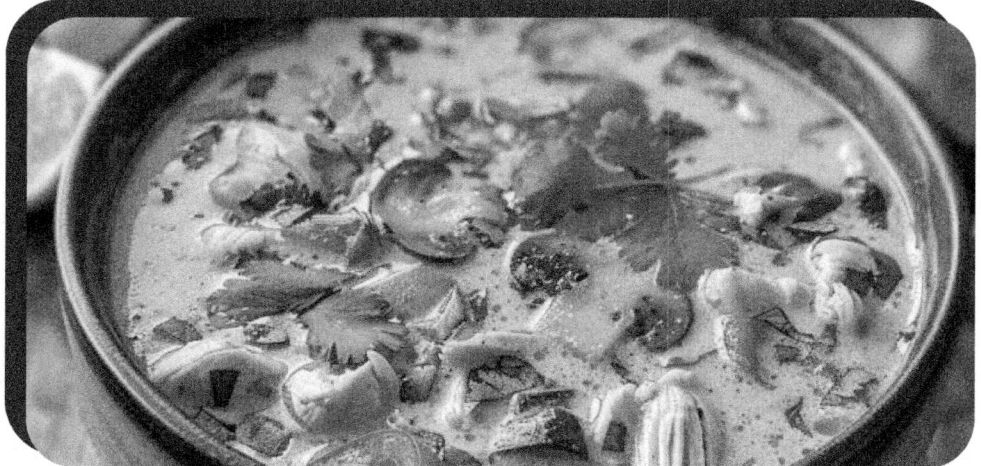

Seafood soup

SERVES 6

- 1 tbsp olive oil
- 1 brown onion, chopped
- 2 carrots, chopped
- 1 green capsicum, chopped
- 1 garlic clove, minced
- 1 bay leaf
- ½ tsp dried oregano
- ¼ tsp dried basil
- ¼ tsp pepper
- 1 400g can diced tomatoes
- 1 410g can tomato puree
- ¾ cup white wine or chicken stock
- 3 tbsp fresh parsley, finely chopped
- 400g salmon fillets, skinned and cut into 3 centimetre cubes
- 500g green prawns, peeled and deveined

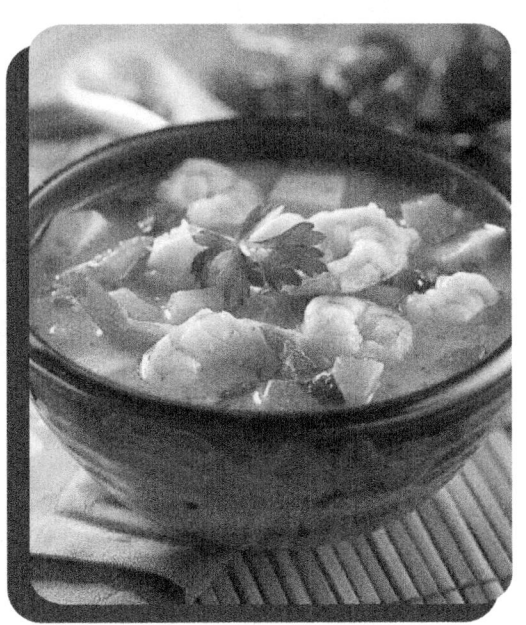

DIRECTIONS

1. Heat oil over medium heat in a large saucepan. Add onion and capsicum and cook, stirring regularly until tender.
2. Add carrots and garlic; cook for 3 minutes before stirring in tomato puree, tomatoes, wine and herbs.
3. Bring to a boil, then reduce heat and simmer, covered, for 30 minutes.
4. Stir in salmon, prawns and parsley.
5. Cook, covered for 10 minutes, or until the fish flakes easily with a fork.
6. Remove bay leaf and if desired, blitz with a food processor until smooth. Serve immediately.

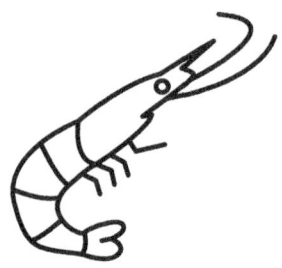
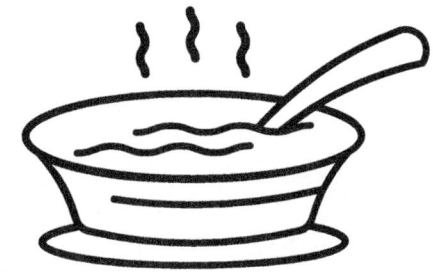

Broccoli and Cashel Blue Soup

SERVES 4

- 28g butter
- 1 large onion, peeled and roughly chopped
- 2 medium potatoes, peeled and diced
- 600ml vegetable or chicken stock
- 420g broccoli
- 250g leek
- 200g celery
- 70g Cashel Blue
- 150ml fresh cream
- Bunch fresh parsley, finely chopped
- Sprig of thyme, finely chopped

DIRECTIONS

1. Place chopped onions in a saucepan with butter, cover with baking paper or foil and sauté while you prepare the potatoes. Add the potatoes to the onions, cover and sauté for a further 2 minutes.
2. Add the stock, bring to a simmer and cook for 5 minutes until potatoes are turning tender, then add chopped broccoli, celery and leeks. Season with salt and pepper. Cook for 5 minutes. Add the fresh herbs, and cook for a further 3 minutes - you are aiming to just cook but still maintain the freshness of the green vegetables.
3. Add fresh cream and Cashel Blue cheese and blend until smooth.
4. Serve immediately with a piece of Cashel Blue added to the top of the soup for extra texture, colour and flavour.

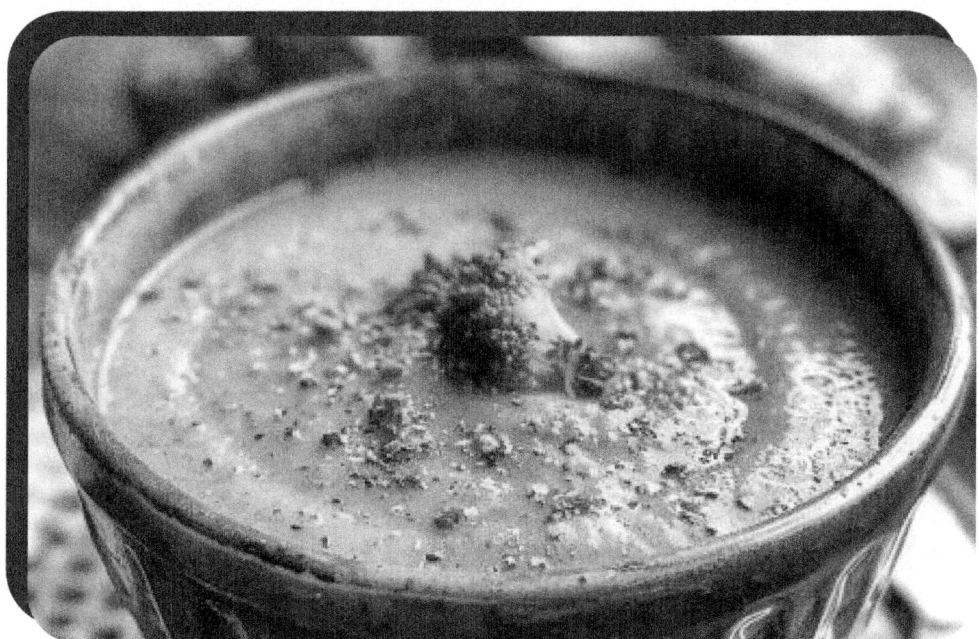

Sweet Corn Soup

SERVES 6

- 6 cobs corns, shucked
- 2 brown onions, 1 quartered and 1 thinly sliced
- 2 ½ centimetre piece of fresh ginger, finely diced
- 3 ¼ litres water, divided
- 1 tbsp coconut oil
- 1 tsp minced ginger
- 4 cloves garlic, minced
- 415 mL coconut milk
- 1 tbsp fresh lime juice
- Salt and pepper

To garnish
- Chilli oil
- Grilled corn kernels

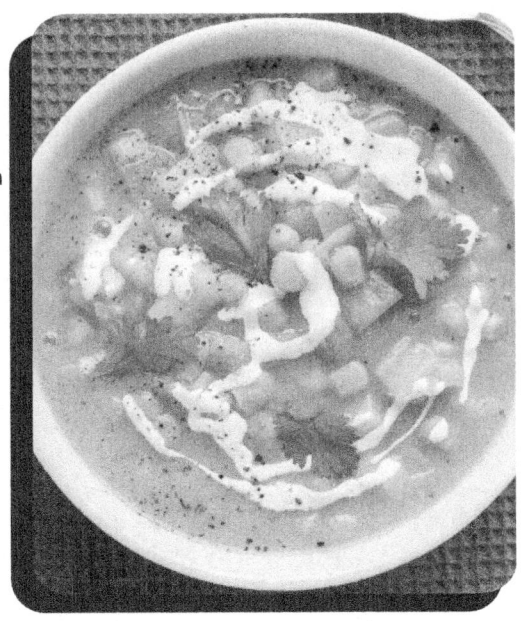

DIRECTIONS

1. Cut kernels from the corn cobs. Set kernels aside and reserve cobs.
2. Add corn cobs, quartered onion, diced ginger and 3 litres of water to a large saucepan and bring to a boil over high heat. Reduce heat and simmer for 1 hour. Strain through a sieve into a large bowl and discard the solids. Set corn stock aside.
3. Heat a medium saucepan over medium-high heat. Add oil, sliced onion, minced ginger, garlic and cook, stirring often for 1 minute, then add remaining water. Reduce heat to medium-low, cover and cook, stirring occasionally until the onion is soft and most of the water has evaporated.
4. Add corn kernels to the saucepan and cook over medium heat, stirring occasionally until the kernels are softened, about 10 minutes. Add reserved corn stock, cover and simmer, stirring occasionally for 30 minutes, then add in coconut milk and simmer for a further 3 minutes.
5. Remove from heat and use a stick blender to blend soup until smooth. Pass soup through a sieve into a clean saucepan. Add lime juice, stir and season to taste.
6. Serve soup hot or cold topped with grilled corn kernels and chilli oil.

Pea Soup with Crispy Pancetta and Parmesan Tuille

SERVES 4

For the Soup
- 2 tbsp olive oil
- 1 large brown onion, roughly chopped
- 2 cloves garlic, sliced
- 1 celery stick, roughly chopped
- 2 medium potatoes, peeled and roughly chopped
- 1 tbsp fresh mint leaves, chopped
- 1 tsp fresh thyme leaves, chopped
- 1 tbsp fresh basil leaves, chopped
- 500 g frozen peas, thawed
- Salt and freshly ground black pepper

Toppings
- 2 cups grated parmesan
- 8 slices pancetta
- Mint and basil leaves

DIRECTIONS

1. Preheat oven to 200C.
2. On a tray lined with baking paper, sprinkle grated parmesan into four rough circles about 8 centimetres wide. Cook in the oven until the cheese melts and turns golden, about 5 minutes. Remove from the oven and shape by bending the cheese over a rolling pin. Set aside to cool.
3. Prepare pancetta by adding slices to a lined baking tray. Cook for 15 minutes or until the pancetta is crisp. Remove from oven and set aside.
4. Meanwhile, heat olive oil in a medium sized saucepan. Add onion, garlic, celery, potatoes, mint, thyme and basil, and sauté for about 5 minutes. Cover with 1 litre of water and bring to a simmer. Reduce heat and gently simmer for 20 minutes or until the vegetables have all softened.
5. Add peas to the saucepan and bring back to the boil. Remove from heat and blend with a stick blender. Taste and season.
6. Add the soup to serving bowls and top with Parmesan tuille, pancetta, and herbs to garnish.

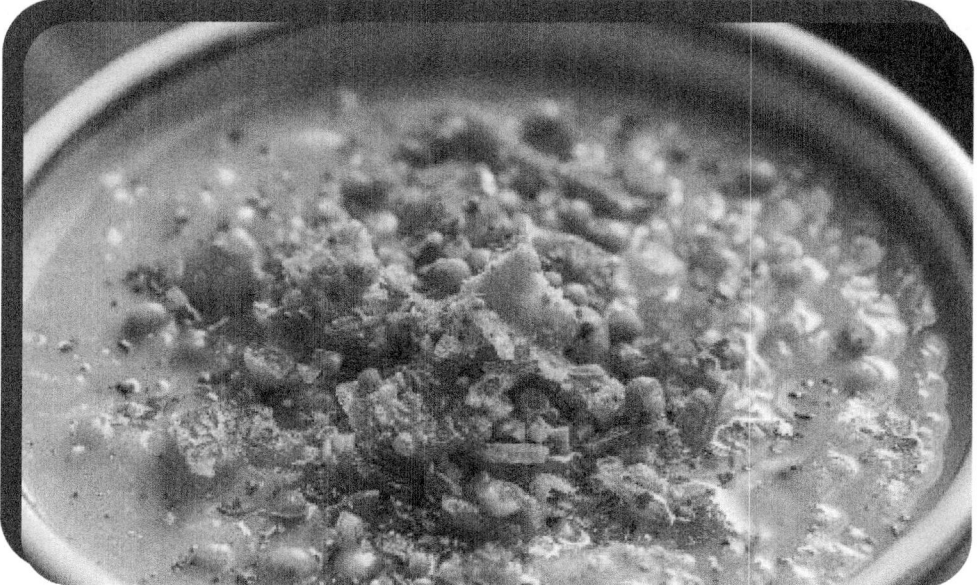

Creamy Cauliflower and Broccoli Soup with Feta

SERVES 4

- 1 tbsp olive oil
- 1 medium brown onion, finely chopped
- 2 cloves garlic, minced
- 3 cups broccoli florets
- 3 cups cauliflower florets
- 2 cups vegetable stock
- 3 cups water
- 1 cup milk
- Salt and pepper to season
- Feta to crumble into soup for serving

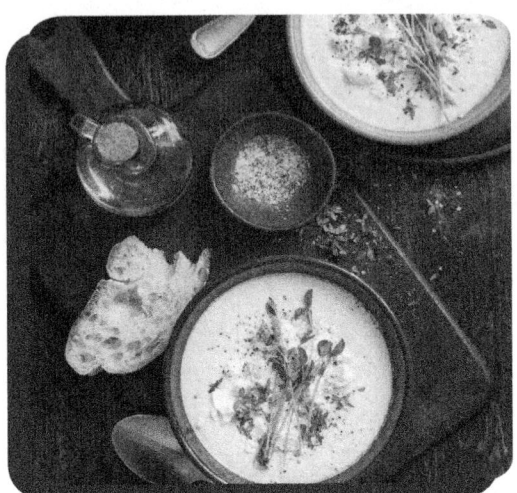

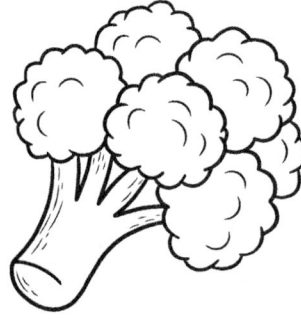

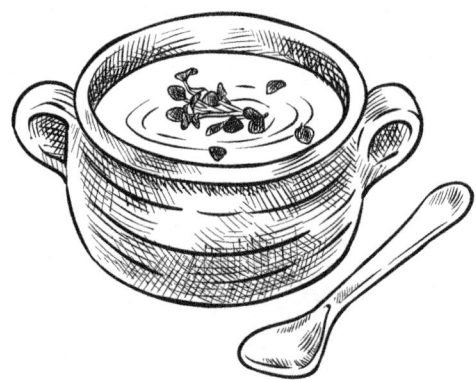

DIRECTIONS

1. Heat olive oil in a large saucepan and add onion and garlic. Cook, stirring constantly until soft.
2. Add cauliflower, broccoli, stock and water and bring to the boil. Reduce heat, cover and simmer for 20 minutes.
3. Remove from heat and blend with a stick blender until smooth. Stir in milk and season with salt and pepper. If the consistency is too thick, add a little more milk or some hot water.
4. Heat gently over low heat until thoroughly warmed.
5. To serve, crumble feta over the soup when it is in bowls.

Mushroom and Parmesan Soup

SERVES 4

- 1 kg button mushrooms
- 2 small brown onions, chopped
- 4 cloves garlic, minced
- 1 tbsp dried Italian seasoning
- Salt, to taste
- Freshly ground black pepper, to taste
- 3 tbsp olive oil, plus extra for drizzling
- ½ cup parmesan cheese, grated, plus extra to serve
- 2 cups vegetable stock, divided
- 2 cups water

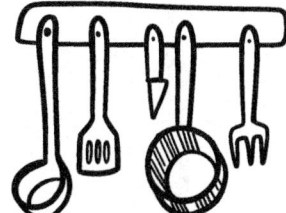

DIRECTIONS

1. Preheat oven to 200C.
2. Add mushrooms, onions, garlic, Italian seasoning, salt, pepper, and olive oil to a large bowl and mix well so that all ingredients are coated in the oil. Tip into a baking tray, spreading out into one layer, and bake for 30 minutes or until the mushrooms are tender. Remove from oven and set aside to cool for 10 minutes, then transfer to a food processor. You may need to work in batches depending on the size of your food processor.
3. Add parmesan cheese and half the vegetable stock to the blender and process until smooth. Transfer to a saucepan set over medium-high heat and add in remaining vegetable stock and water. Stir well and cook until the soup is heated throughout, then serve drizzled with a little olive oil and a garnished with parmesan, salt and a good crack of black pepper.

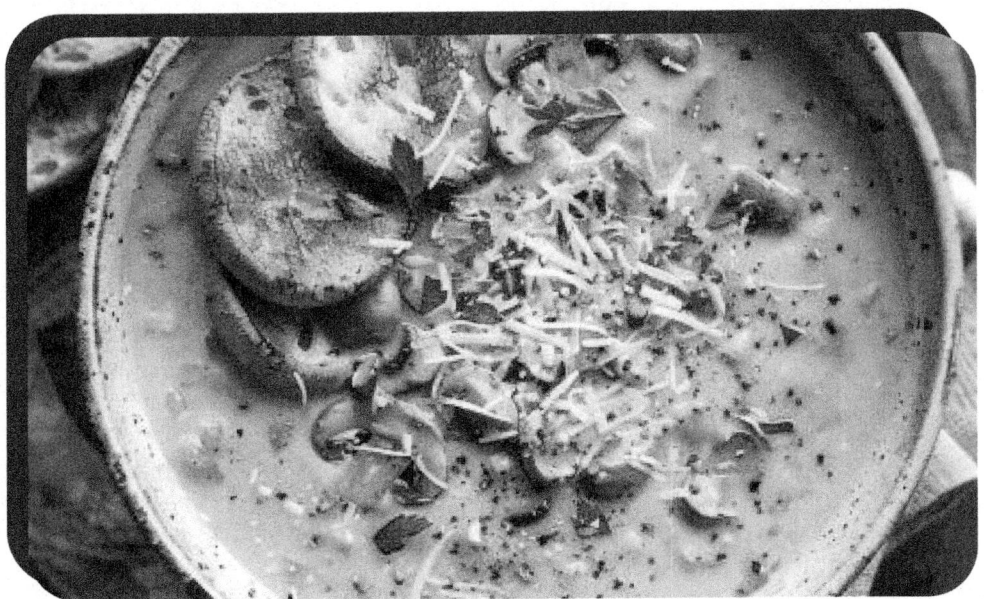

Oyster Soup

SERVES 6

- 5 tbsp unsalted butter
- 2 dozen oysters
- ¼ cup plain flour
- 2 stalks celery, finely diced
- 1 brown onion, finely diced
- 1 ¾ cups milk
- ¼ cup cream
- Salt
- Freshly ground black pepper
- Tabasco sauce (optional)

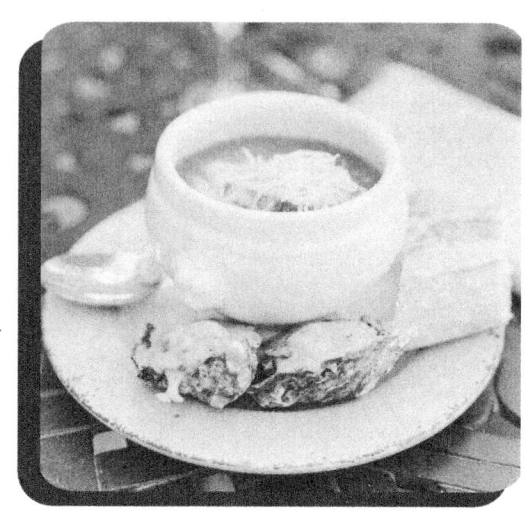

DIRECTIONS

1. Remove oysters from their shells and place in a bowl.
2. Melt butter in a saucepan over medium heat. Add flour and stir vigorously, then reduce heat to low and cook for 2-3 minutes, stirring constantly, until it is a pale tan colour.
3. Add celery and onions and increase heat to medium and cook for 2 minutes, stirring frequently, then slowly add the milk and cream, stirring constantly. Season to taste and if you would like a little spice, add Tabasco to taste.
4. Reduce heat to very low, ensuring the soup does not boil and cook for 15 minutes.
5. Add oysters and cook for 2 minutes or until the edges of the oysters just start to curl. You can choose to puree the soup if you would prefer a smooth texture or otherwise serve as is, topped with a piece of crusty baguette and a little grated parmesan cheese.

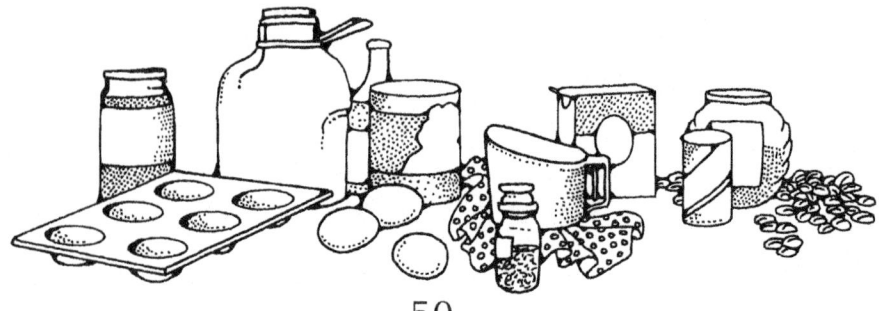

Harissa-Spiced Creamy Tomato Soup

SERVES 4

- 3 tbsp olive oil, divided
- 1 brown onion, chopped
- 3 cloves garlic, minced
- 1 tsp paprika
- ½ tsp cumin
- 2 x 400g tins chopped or whole tomatoes
- 2 tbsp Herbie's Harissa Paste Mix
- 2 tsp honey
- 1 x 400ml tin coconut milk
- 150g chickpeas, drained and rinsed
- Salt and pepper to taste
- ¼ cup coriander (optional, to serve)
- 100g goat cheese, crumbled (optional, to serve)

DIRECTIONS

1. Make a harissa paste by combining 2 tablespoons of Harissa Paste Mix with 2 tablespoons of water. Mix and set aside.
2. In a large pan over medium heat, add 1 tablespoon olive oil. Add chickpeas and a pinch of salt. Cook, stirring until the chickpeas are golden and crispy, about 5 minutes. Remove chickpeas from pan and set aside.
3. Using the same pan, heat remaining 2 tablespoons of olive oil over medium heat. Add onion, garlic and a pinch each of salt and pepper. Cook until onion is beginning to caramelise. Add paprika and cumin and cook for another minute. Add tomatoes, harissa mix and honey and cook for a further 5 minutes, stirring with a wooden spoon and using the spoon to break up the tomatoes.
4. Remove from heat and add coconut milk. Use a stick blender to blend until almost smooth. Return to low heat and gently simmer. Taste and season if needed. If soup is too thick, thin with more coconut milk or a little water.
5. Serve soup with crispy chickpeas and coriander and goat cheese if desired.

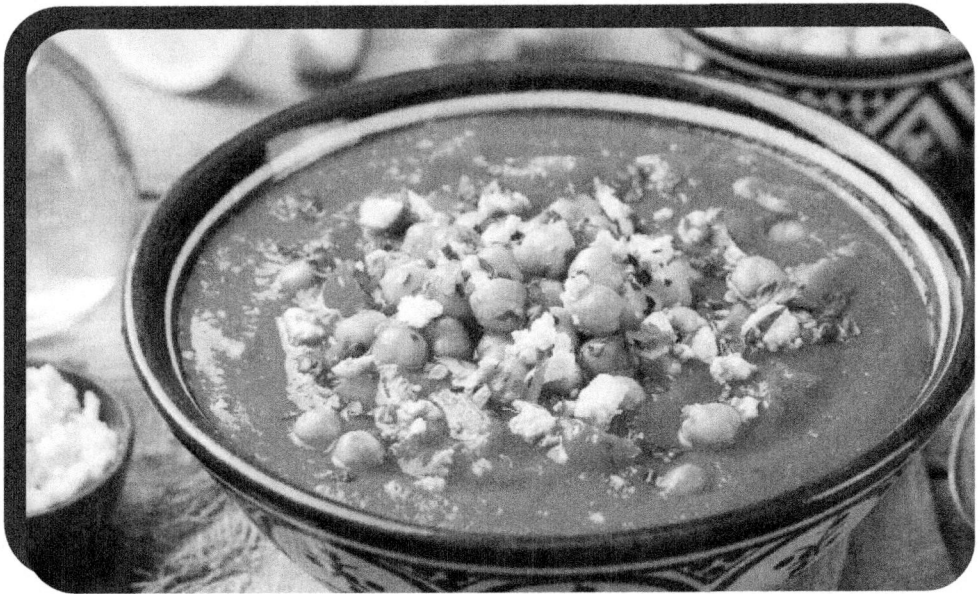

Japanese ramen turkey noodle soup

SERVES 4

- 700 ml chicken stock
- 3 cloves garlic, crushed
- 4 tbsp soy sauce
- 2 cm piece of ginger, sliced
- ½ tsp Chinese five spice
- Pinch of chilli powder
- 300 ml water
- 2 tbsp sesame oil
- 250 g extra firm tofu
- 375 g ramen noodles
- 400 g cooked turkey, sliced
- 100 g mushrooms, thinly sliced
- 4 boiled eggs, peeled and halved
- 100 g baby spinach leaves

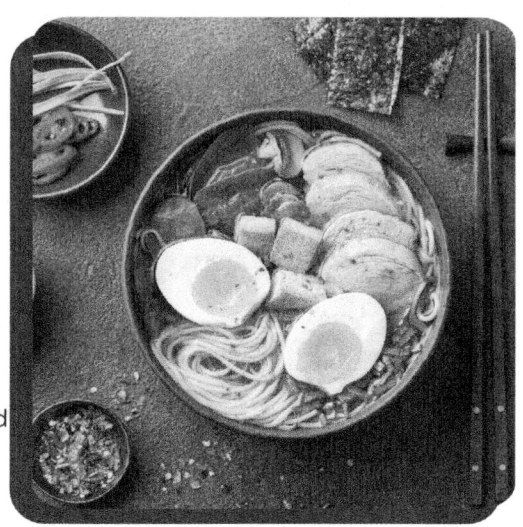

DIRECTIONS

1. Add chicken stock, garlic, soy sauce, ginger, Chinese five spice, chilli powder and water in a large saucepan and bring to the boil, then reduce heat and simmer for 5 minutes.
2. Press as much moisture as you can out of the tofu and cut into cubes. Heat sesame oil over medium high heat and cook tofu until it is browned.
3. Cook noodles according to the packet instructions, drain and set aside.
4. Slice turkey and set aside.
5. Divide noodles between 4 bowls, top each with one-quarter each of the turkey, mushrooms, spinach and tofu and two boiled egg halves.
6. Strain stock into a clean pan and bring to the boil again.
7. Divide stock between bowls and serve immediately.

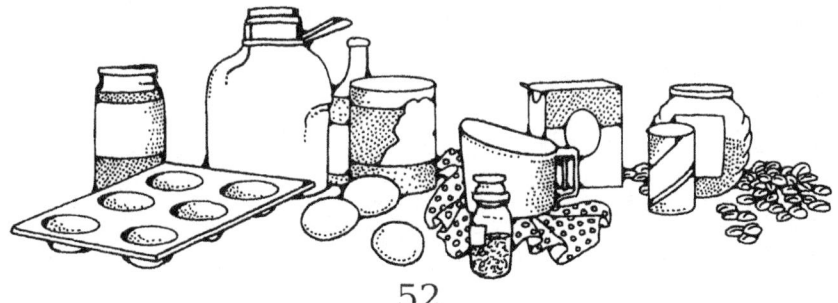

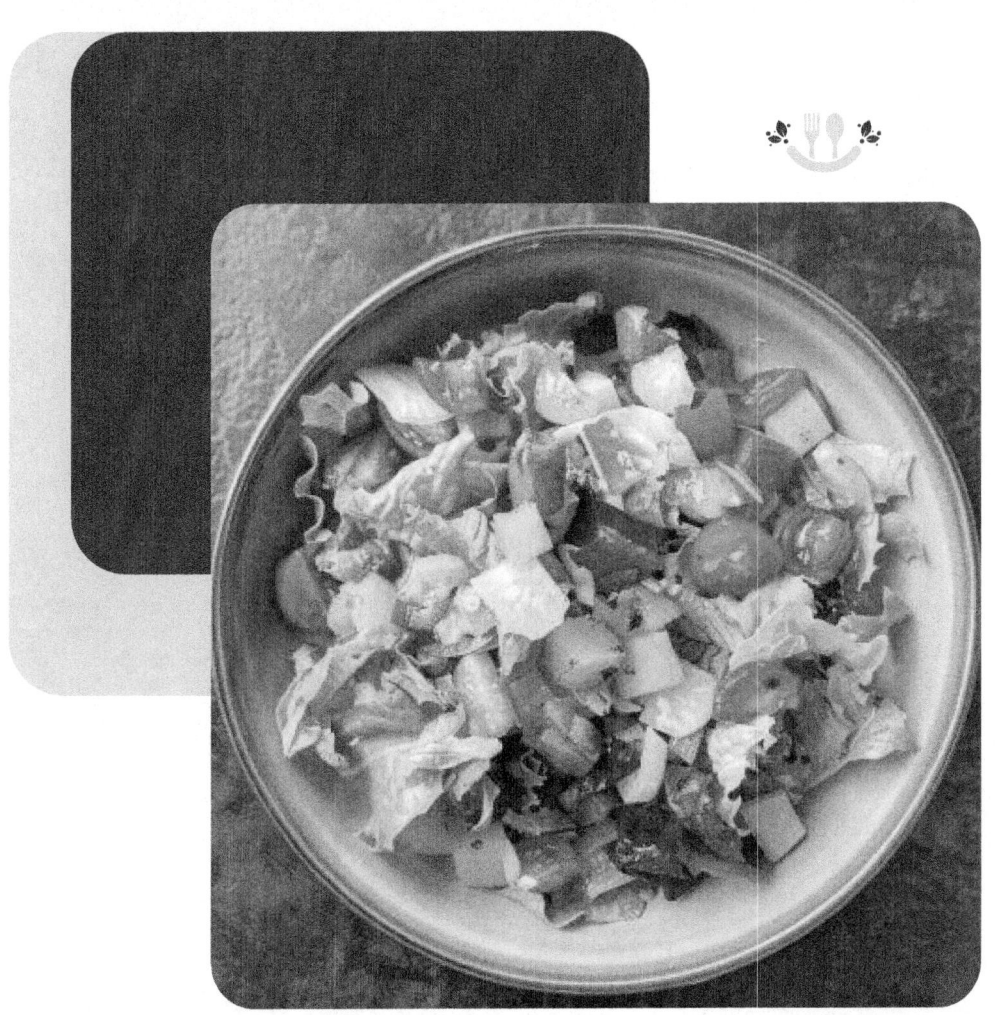

Salad

Salad is a dish usually made from fresh vegetables, chopped and mixed with a variety of ingredients such as fruits, nuts, cheese, meat or seafood. Salads are often eaten with a sauce or cooking oil to enhance the flavor. Salad can be served as an appetizer, a main dish, or as a side dish depending on the ingredients and preparation. Salads are not only popular because of their convenience and ease of preparation, but they are also a healthy choice thanks to their high vitamin and mineral content from vegetables and fruits.

Cobb Salad

SERVES 6

For the Dressing
- 1/3 cup red wine vinegar
- 1 tbsp Dijon mustard
- 2/3 cup olive oil
- 1 garlic clove, minced
- Salt to taste
- Freshly ground black pepper to taste

For the Salad
- 8 rashers bacon, roughly chopped
- 4 large free range eggs
- 1 cos lettuce, roughly chopped
- 3 cups barbecue chicken, chopped
- 3 tomatoes, quartered
- 1 avocado, peeled and diced
- 125 g blue cheese, crumbled

DIRECTIONS

1. Add dressing ingredients to a jar and shake well to combine. Set aside.
2. Preheat oven to 200C. Line a baking tray with baking paper and lay bacon on the tray. Cook in oven for 10 minutes, then flip pieces and return to the oven for a further 5 minutes or until the bacon is well cooked and starting to crisp.
3. Meanwhile place eggs in a saucepan and cover with cold water (you should fill the pan to approximately 1 centimetre above the eggs. Cook over high heat until the water comes to the boil. When the water is boiling, remove from saucepan from the heat and cover with a lid. Leave for 6 minutes before removing eggs and placing in a bowl of iced water to cool for 10 minutes. When eggs have cooled, remove the shell and cut them into quarters.
4. Arrange lettuce on a platter and then add rows of chicken, bacon, avocado, tomato and avocado.
5. When ready to serve, shake the dressing and drizzle over salad, before crumbling blue cheese on the top.

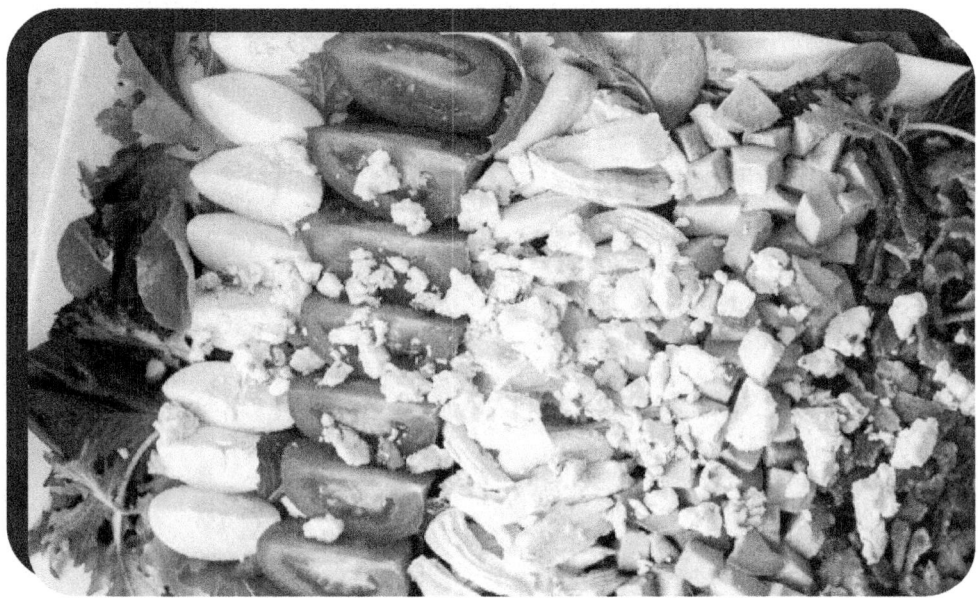

Instant Noodle Vegetable Salad

SERVES 4

- 2 packets instant noodles
- 2 cups shredded red cabbage
- 1 cup broccoli florets
- 1 large carrot, peeled and cut into matchsticks
- ½ red capsicum, diced
- ½ yellow capsicum, diced
- 1 cup sugar snap peas
- 1 spring onion, green part only, sliced
- ¼ cup peanuts, chopped

For the dressing

- 1/3 cup vegetable oil
- ¼ cup rice wine vinegar
- 1 tbsp sugar
- Seasoning from noodle packets

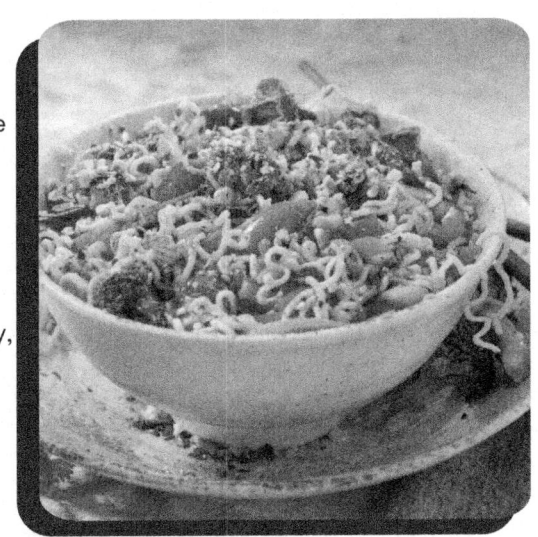

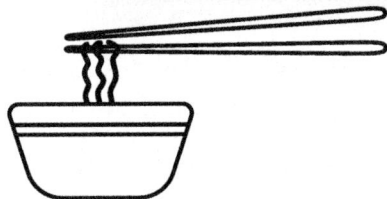

DIRECTIONS

1. Remove noodles from the packets and place in a large bowl, setting aside the seasoning packets.
2. Fill kettle and put on to boil. When kettle has boiled pour boiling water over the noodles to cover them completely. Allow to sit for 1 minute, then use a fork to separate noodles. Leave noodles in the boiling water until they are soft, then drain and place in the fridge to cool.
3. Meanwhile, place broccoli in a microwave-safe bowl with 3 tablespoons of water and cover with a lid or a plate. Microwave on high for 2 ½ minutes or until the broccoli is tender but still holding its shape. Remove from microwave and set aside.
4. When noodles have cooled add to a large bowl with shredded red cabbage, broccoli, carrot, yellow and red capsicum, sugar snap peas, and spring onion. Toss to combine all ingredients.
5. Add all dressing ingredients to a small bowl and whisk to combine.
6. Pour dressing over salad and toss to coat. Serve garnished with chopped peanuts.

Tuscan Panzanella with Peaches

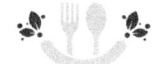

SERVES 4 AS A SIDE SALAD

- 4 cups day-old bread, cut into 2 ½ centimetre pieces
- 1 tbsp olive oil
- 200 g of assorted cherry tomatoes, halved
- 1 tsp salt
- 2 Lebanese cucumbers, cut into 2 ½ centimetre pieces
- 1 large red onion, sliced
- 1 cup basil leaves
- 2 yellow peaches, pitted, grilled, and sliced
- 100 g buffalo mozzarella, torn

For the dressing

- 2 tbsp white wine vinegar
- 1 tsp Dijon mustard
- 8 tbsp olive oil
- 2 cloves garlic, minced
- Generous pinch of salt

DIRECTIONS

1. Preheat oven to 180C.
2. Pour olive oil in a bowl and add bread. Toss to coat. Spread bread onto a baking tray and cook for 15 minutes, or until golden brown. Remove from oven and set aside.
3. Meanwhile prepare salad by adding tomatoes, to a strainer or colander set over a bowl. Sprinkle tomatoes with salt and leave for 10 minutes to draw out juices.
4. Add cucumber, red onion, basil and peaches to a large bowl. Add tomatoes and reserve tomato juice for the dressing. Toss tomatoes, cucumber, red onion, basil and peaches together gently.
5. Make the dressing by adding white wine vinegar, mustard, olive oil, garlic and salt to the bowl with the reserved tomato juice and whisk well.
6. To serve, add cooled bread to the salad and toss, then pour over dressing and toss again. Wait a few minutes to allow the juices to soak into the bread, then add torn mozzarella and serve.

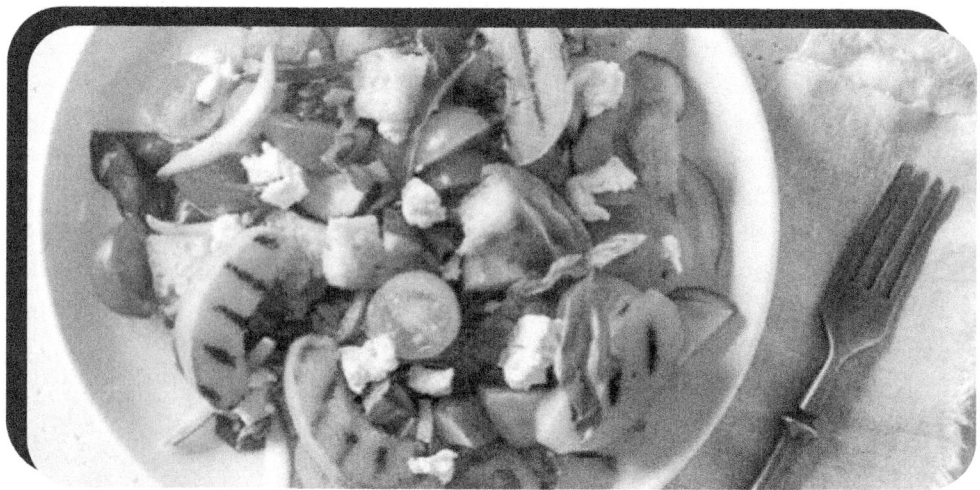

Tabbouleh Salad with Cauliflower Rice and Vegetables

SERVES 4 AS A SIDE DISH

- 1 large cauliflower
- 1 medium cucumber, chopped
- 175 g cherry tomatoes, halved
- 3 spring onions, chopped
- 1/3 cup mint leaves, chopped
- 1/3 cup flat leaf parsley leaves, chopped
- Zest of ½ lemon
- Lemon wedges to serve

For the dressing

- ¼ cup lemon juice
- 1 tbsp red wine vinegar
- 2 tbsp olive oil
- 1 clove garlic, minced
- Salt
- Freshly ground black pepper

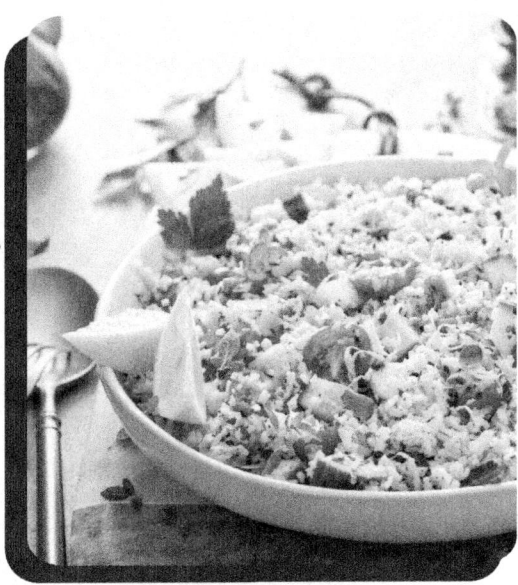

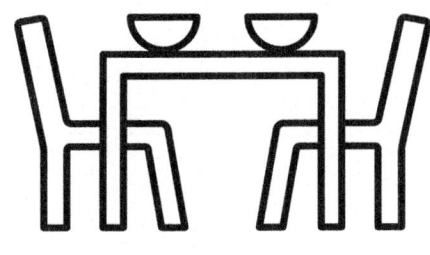

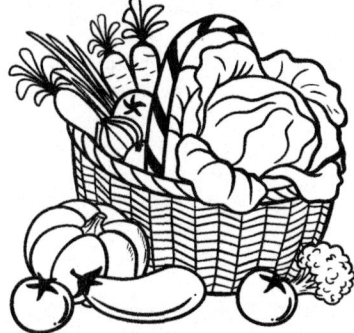

DIRECTIONS

1. Cut cauliflower into large pieces and place in a food processor. If using a food processor, attach the grater attachment and grate into rice. If using a box grater, grate until pieces are the size of grains of rice. If using a knife, continue chopping until the cauliflower is finely chopped into rice-sized pieces.
2. Add cauliflower rice to a large bowl, then add cucumber, tomatoes, onion, mint, parsley, and lemon zest and toss to combine.
3. Whisk dressing ingredients together and season to taste. Pour dressing over cauliflower rice and vegetables and toss again.
4. Serve immediately with lemon wedges or store in the fridge before serving.

Curried Cauliflower Salad

SERVES 6

- 1 cauliflower, chopped into small florets
- 400 g can of chickpeas, drained
- ½ tsp turmeric
- 1 tsp smoked paprika
- ½ tsp ground ginger
- ½ tsp chilli powder
- ½ tsp table salt
- Olive oil
- 150 g baby spinach leaves
- 100 g pine nuts
- ½ bunch mint leaves, chopped
- ½ bunch coriander leaves, chopped, plus extra for garnish
- 100 g pomegranate aril

For the Dressing
- 150 g Greek yoghurt
- 3 tbsp mango chutney
- 1 lime
- Pinch of salt

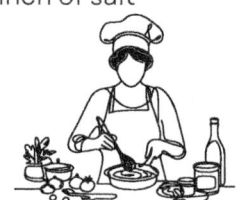

DIRECTIONS

1. Preheat oven to 180C.
2. Add cauliflower and chickpeas to a baking tray. Combine turmeric, paprika, ginger, chilli powder and salt in a small bowl. Pour spices over cauliflower and chickpeas and toss to coat. Drizzle generously with olive oil and toss again.
3. Cook for 15-20 minutes or until cauliflower is almost cooked. Add spinach leaves and pine nuts, and cook for a further 8 minutes.
4. Remove from the oven and set aside to cool.
5. Meanwhile make the dressing by adding yoghurt and chutney to a bowl with the zest and juice of the lime, and a pinch of salt. Mix well.
6. When the cauliflower has cooled, add mint, coriander, and pomegranate, and toss to combine.
7. Serve topped with dressing and garnished with extra coriander leaves.

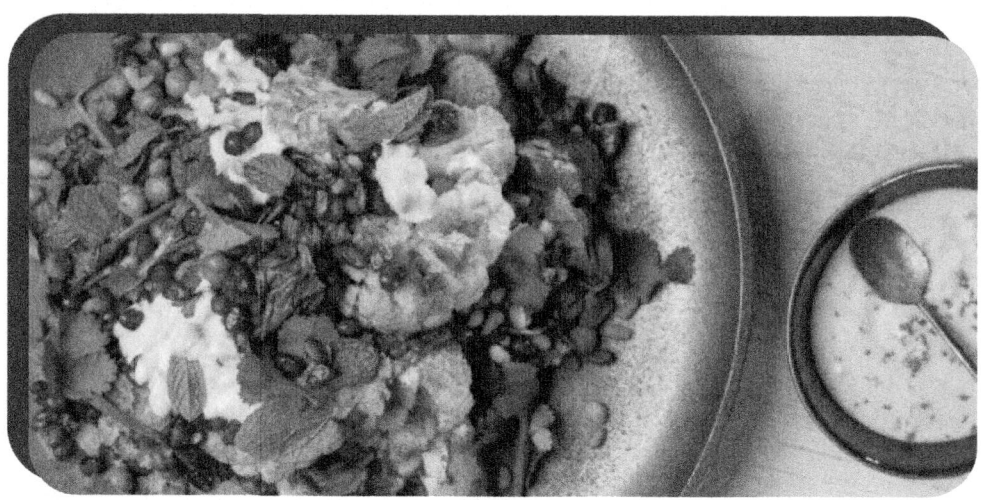

Watermelon and Cucumber Salad with Feta and Mint

SERVES 4

- ½ large watermelon, cut into cubes
- 1 continental cucumber, cut in half lengthways, then cut into half-rounds
- 1 large handful of mint leaves
- ½ cup feta, crumbled
- 3 tbsp olive oil
- 1 tbsp lime juice
- Salt, to taste
- Freshly cracked black pepper, to taste

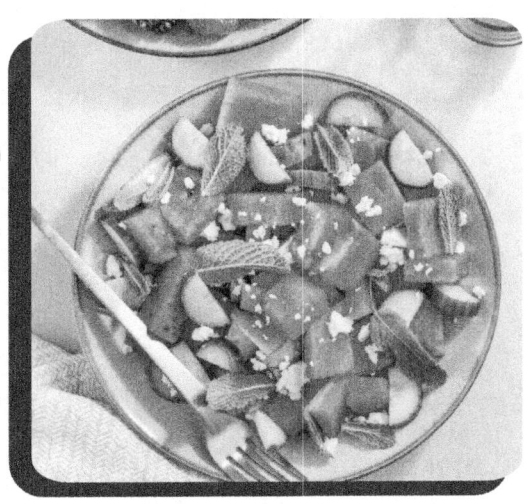

DIRECTIONS

1. Add watermelon, cucumber and mint to a large bowl.
2. Mix olive oil and lime juice together in a small bowl and season to taste.
3. Pour dressing over the watermelon mixture and toss to coat well.
4. Crumble feta over the top and serve immediately.

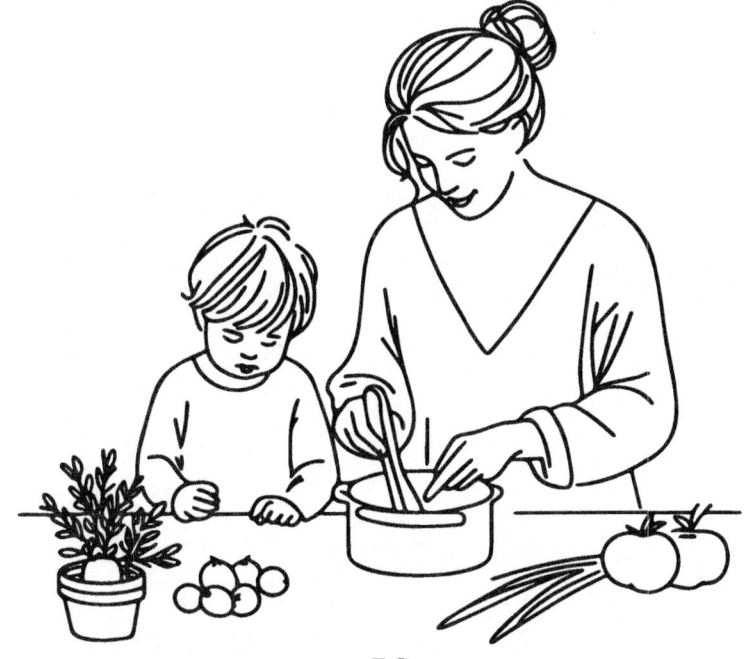

Roasted Sweet Potato and Black Bean Salad

SERVES 4

- 1 kg sweet potatoes, peeled and diced
- 6 tbsp olive oil
- 1 ½ tsp salt
- Freshly ground black pepper
- ¼ cup raw pumpkin seeds
- 1 tsp chilli flakes
- Juice of 2 limes
- 400 g can black beans
- 1 small red onion, peeled and chopped
- 1 large avocado, peeled and chopped
- 1 handful coriander, chopped
- 2 spring onions, chopped

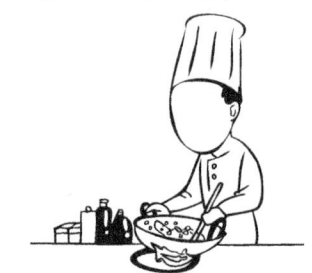

DIRECTIONS

1. Preheat oven to 200C.
2. Pour 1 tbsp of olive oil onto a baking tray and add sweet potatoes. Add another 2 tbsp oil, along with the salt and a couple of generous grinds of black pepper. Arrange sweet potato evenly in the tray and roast for 20 minutes, then turn and roast for a further 10 minutes, or until the sweet potato is tender and golden.
3. Meanwhile add pumpkin seeds and remaining olive oil to a frying pan over medium heat. Cook, watching closely for 2 minutes or until the pumpkin seeds are starting to change colour, then remove from the heat and season with salt and chilli flakes. Set aside.
4. Remove sweet potatoes from the oven and pour over pumpkin seeds and olive oil mix. Pour over lime juice.
5. Drain and rinse black beans and add them to the tray. Add red onion, avocado, coriander and spring onions and toss to combine.
6. Spoon salad into a serving bowl and serve warm or cold.

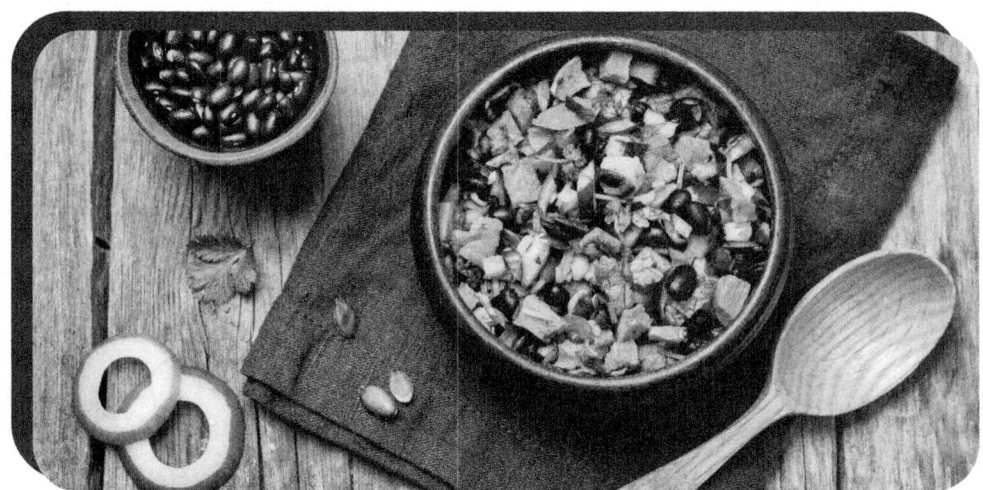

Truss Tomato Salad with Duo of Basil

SERVES 6

- 8 truss tomatoes, sliced
- 1 bunch purple basil
- Olive oil
- Salt
- 150 g bocconcini balls
- Freshly ground black pepper

For the Basil Oil
- ½ cup olive oil
- 1 cup tightly packed basil leaves
- Pinch of salt

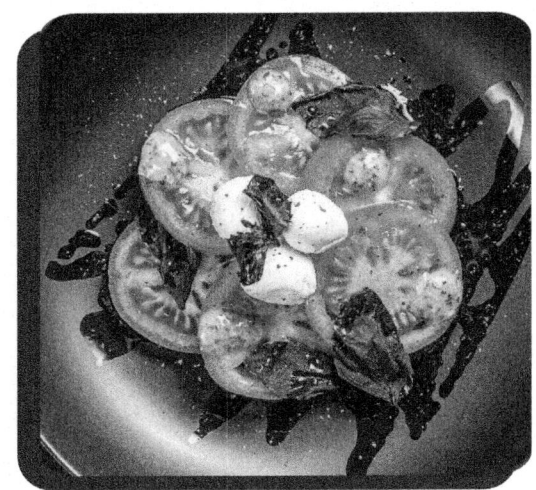

DIRECTIONS

1. Line a baking tray with baking paper.
2. Rinse purple basil leaves well and pat dry between two sheets of paper towel or two clean tea towels. Lay the basil leaves on the baking tray and spritz with olive oil or cooking spray and sprinkle with sea salt. Bake for 5 to 8 minutes or until crispy. Remove from oven and allow to cool.
3. Make Basil Oil by blanching basil leaves in a pot of boiling water for 10 seconds. Remove, strain and dunk in ice water. Remove from water and squeeze to remove excess water. Add leaves to a food processor with olive oil and a pinch of salt. Blend until the basil is pureed. Strain to remove any solids and set aside.
4. To serve, drizzle plates with olive oil and arrange tomatoes on top. Add bocconcini balls and dollop basil oil on top of tomatoes. Lay purple basil chips on plate and finish with a grind of black pepper.

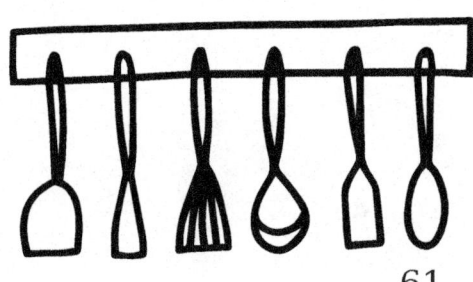
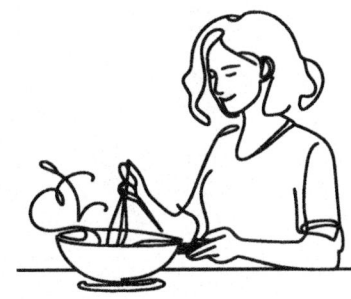

Good for You Salad

SERVES 4

- ½ large butternut pumpkin, peeled and cut into approximately 1 ½ centimetre cubes
- ¼ cup olive oil, plus 2 tablespoons, divided
- 1 x 400 g can chickpeas, drained
- 1 apple, cored and sliced
- 50 g pepitas
- 50 g dried cranberries
- 1 tbsp lemon juice
- 1 tsp maple syrup
- Pinch each of salt and freshly ground black pepper

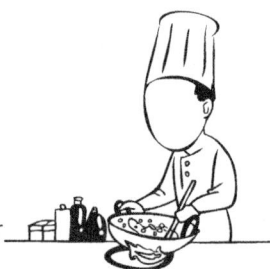

DIRECTIONS

1. Preheat oven to 180C.
2. Add pumpkin and 2 tablespoons olive oil to a roasting pan and season with salt and pepper. Roast for 30 minutes.
3. Wash and roughly chop the kale and add to a serving bowl. Add chickpeas, apple, pepitas, cranberries and pumpkin.
4. Add remaining olive oil, lemon juice and maple syrup to a small bowl with salt and pepper and whisk to combine.
5. Pour dressing over the salad immediately before serving.

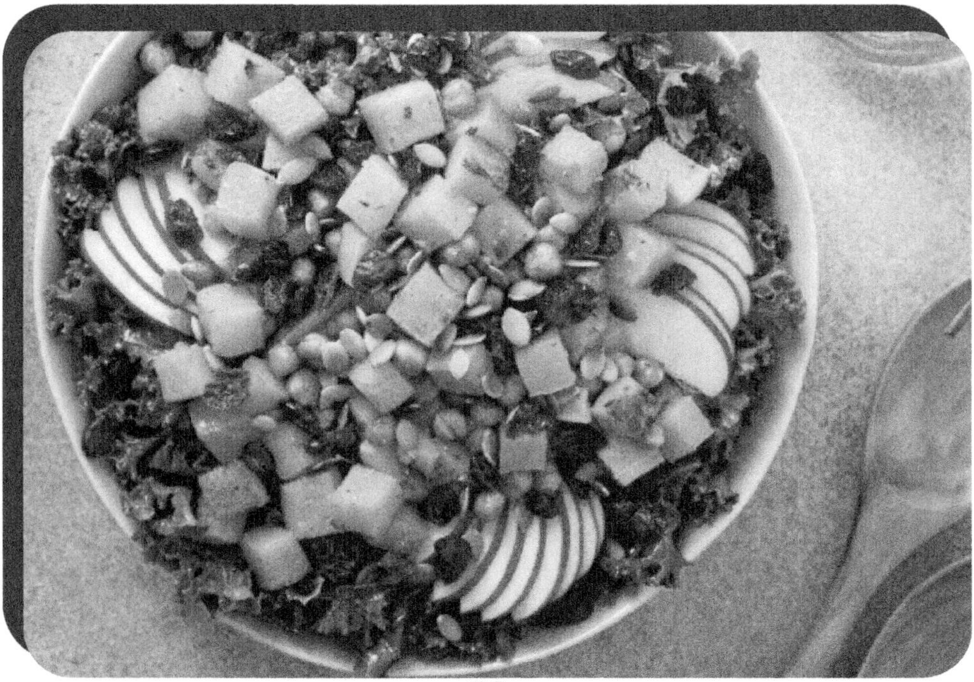

Green Veggie Buddha Bowl

SERVES 6

- 200 g quinoa or other grain of your choice, cooked according to packet directions
- 1 tbsp olive oil
- 250 g broccoli florets
- 2 bunches asparagus
- 2 cups baby spinach
- 2 cups rocket
- 1 cucumber, thinly sliced
- 2 Granny Smith apples, cored and sliced
- 2 avocados, pitted and sliced

For the Dressing

- 1 cup Greek yoghurt
- 1 cup fresh green herbs of your choice, try coriander, parsley, dill, basil, or mint
- ¼ cup spring onion, sliced
- 1 clover garlic, chopped
- Pinch of salt
- Freshly ground black pepper, to taste

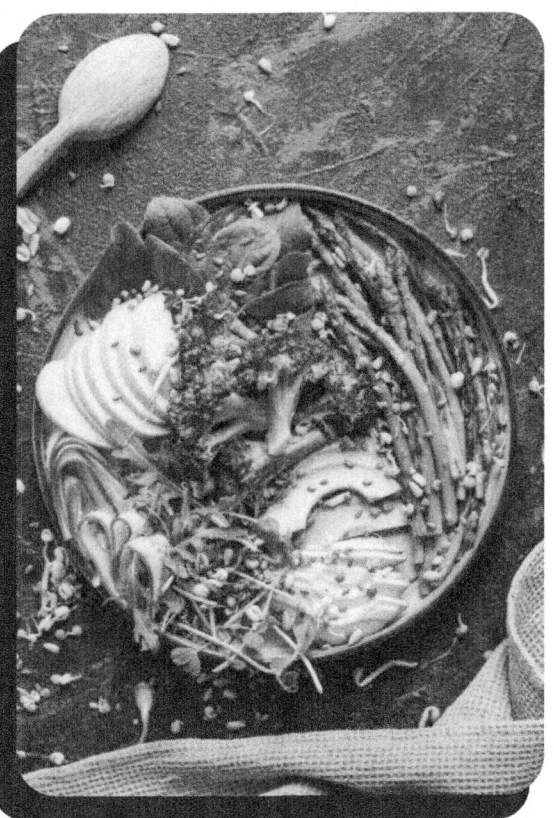

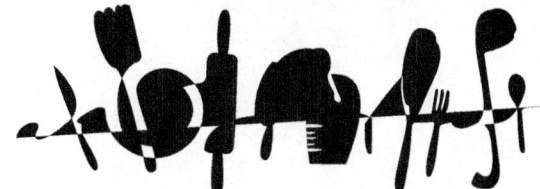

DIRECTIONS

1. Heat oil in a large frying pan over medium-high heat. Toss in broccoli and asparagus and saute for 2 minutes, stirring. Add 3 tablespoons of water, cover the frying pan and steam for 5 minutes.
2. Divide cooked grain between bowls, and top with remaining ingedients.
3. Make dressing by adding all ingredients to a blender and blitzing until creamy.
4. Serve Bowl with dressing.

Plum, Beet, and Pecan Salad

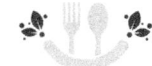

SERVES 4 AS A SIDE SALAD

- 4 beetroot, about tennis ball size
- 6 plums, cut into wedges
- 80 g pecans, toasted and roughly chopped
- ½ bunch mint, leaves
- 1 ½ tbsp olive oil
- ½ tbsp red wine vinegar
- ½ tbsp pomegranate molasses

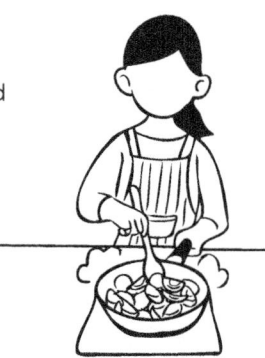

DIRECTIONS

1. Preheat oven to 200C.
2. Remove any leaves from beetroot, leaving a 2 ½ centimetre stem. Rinse beetroot under cold running water and then wrap each beetroot loosely in aluminium foil. Place in a limed baking tray and cook for 45 – 60 minutes or until they are knife tender. Remove from oven and set aside to cool a little in the foil.
3. While the beetroot are warm, use a sharp knife to trim the stem and root ends and to peel the skin from the beetroot. Cut beetroot into wedges.
4. Add beetroot, plums, pecans, and three-quarters of the mint to a bowl.
5. Mix olive oil, red wine vinegar and pomegranate molasses in a small bowl and pour over the salad and toss to coat.
6. Garnish with remaining mint and serve.

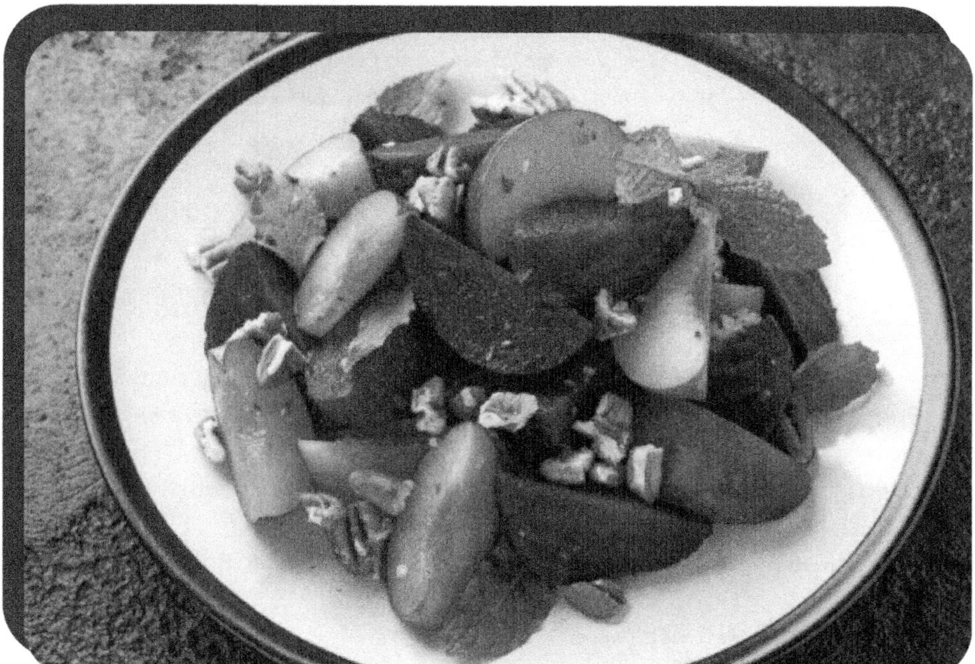

Quinoa Ribbon Salad

SERVES 4

- 2 cups cooked quinoa
- 1 cucumber, shaved into ribbons
- 1 carrot, shaved into ribbons
- 2 cups baby spinach leaves
- 1 cup sugar snap or snow peas
- 60 g pomegranate arils
- 1/3 cup olive oil
- 1 tbsp red wine vinegar
- Juice of 1 lemon
- Juice of 1 lime
- Salt, to taste
- Freshly ground black pepper, to taste
- Lime wedges, to garnish

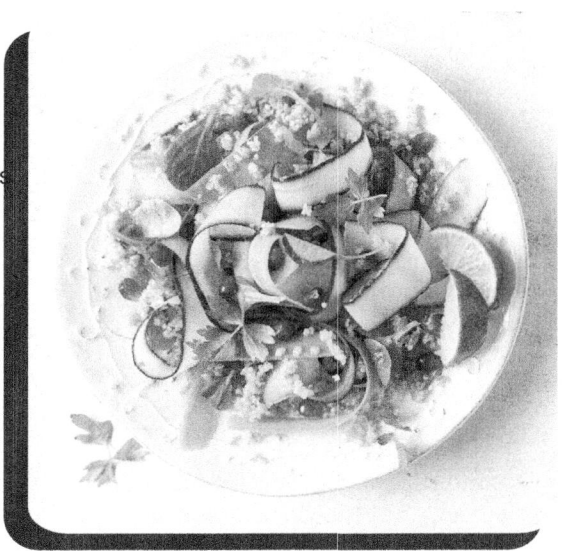

DIRECTIONS

1. Add quinoa to a large bowl with vegetables and pomegranate arils.
2. Add olive oil, red wine vinegar, lemon juice, and lime juice to a small bowl and whisk to combine. Taste, and season.
3. Pour dressing over salad and serve immediately.

TOP TIPS: Dressing can be prepared up to 4 days in advance and stored in an airtight container in the fridge. Shake well before using.

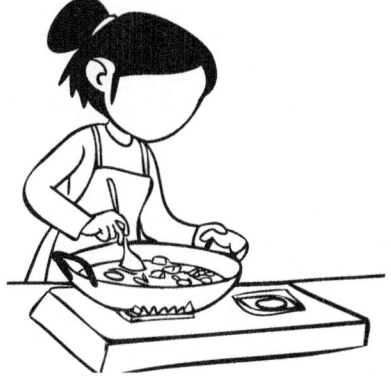
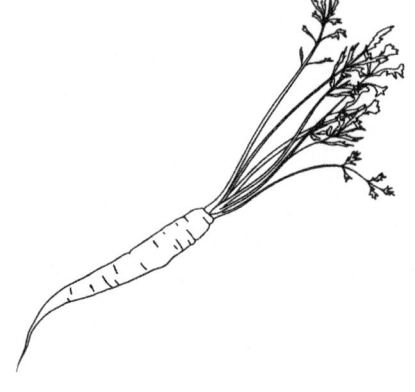

Cucumber, Radish, and Green Pea Salad

SERVES 6

- 6 large iceberg lettuce leaves, torn
- A large handful of rocket leaves, torn
- 4 radishes, finely sliced
- 1 continental cucumber, thinly sliced
- 250 g freshly shelled peas
- Half a bunch of fresh dill, leaves picked

For the Dressing
- 1/3 cup sour cream
- 4 tbsp water
- 2 tbsp fresh dill, chopped
- 1 tbsp olive oil
- 1 tbsp lemon juice
- ½ tsp salt
- ¼ tsp freshly ground black pepper

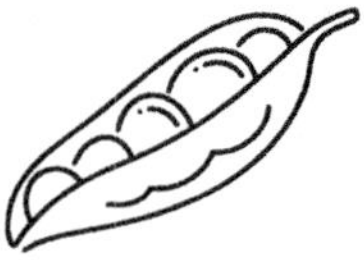

DIRECTIONS

1. Combine lettuce, rocket, radishes, cucumber, peas, and dill leaves in a large bowl.
2. Mix sour cream, water, 2 tablespoons dill, olive oil, lemon juice, salt, and pepper in a small bowl and whisk.
3. Pour dressing over salad and toss to coat. Serve immediately.

TOP TIPS: If fresh peas are not available, you can replace with cooked and chilled frozen peas, or drained canned peas.

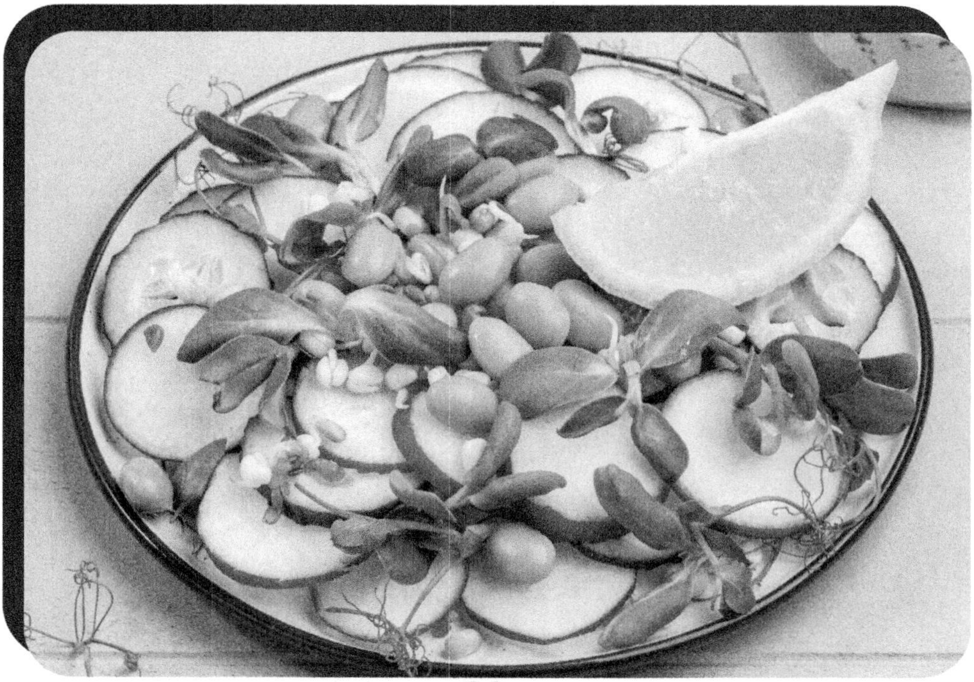

Watermelon Salad with Halloumi and Mint

SERVES 6

- 250 g halloumi, thinly sliced
- 1 ½ tbsp olive oil, divided
- 1 kg watermelon flesh, cut into triangles
- Bunch of mint, roughly chopped
- 1 ½ tbsp balsamic vinegar
- Salt
- Freshly ground black pepper

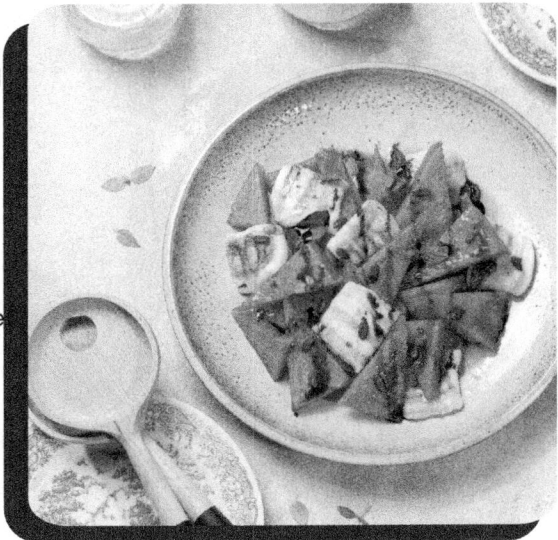

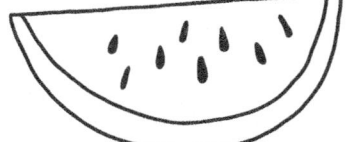

DIRECTIONS

1. Heat barbecue or grill pan over high heat.
2. Lay halloumi on a baking tray and lightly oil with ½ tablespoon olive oil, then grill for 2 minutes per side or until golden.
3. Add watermelon to a bowl with mint, balsamic, and 1 tablespoon olive oil. Season with salt and pepper, then gently toss to combine.
4. Arrange watermelon on a serving plate with halloumi and serve

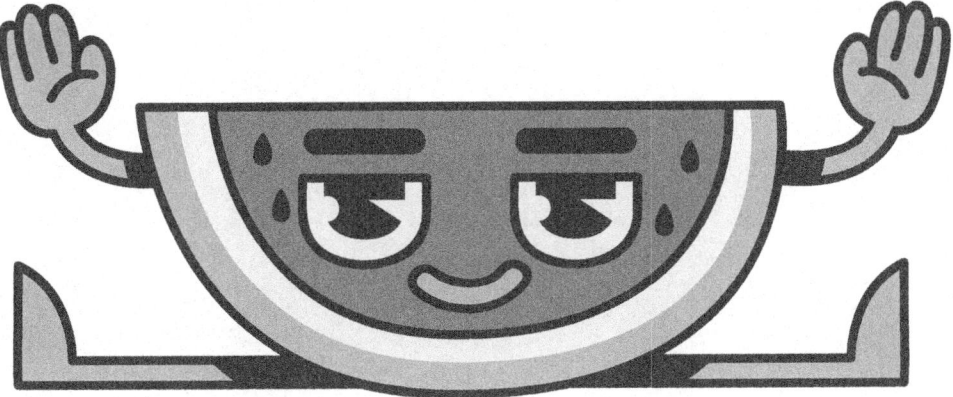

Chicken Waldorf Salad

SERVES 4

For the dressing
- ½ cup mayonnaise
- 2 tbsp wholegrain mustard
- Juice of ½ lemon

For the salad
- 2 ½ cups cold chicken, roughly chopped
- 5 sticks celery, chopped
- 2 apples, cored and chopped
- 1 ½ cups red seedless grapes, cut into halves
- 1 ¼ cup walnuts, roughly chopped, divided
- Salt, to taste
- Pepper, to taste

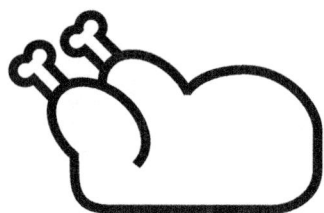

DIRECTIONS

1. Add dressing ingredients to a bowl and whisk to combine. Set aside.
2. Add chicken, celery, apples, grapes and 1 cup walnuts to a large bowl, pour over dressing and toss well to coat.
3. Serve on plates and top with reserved walnuts

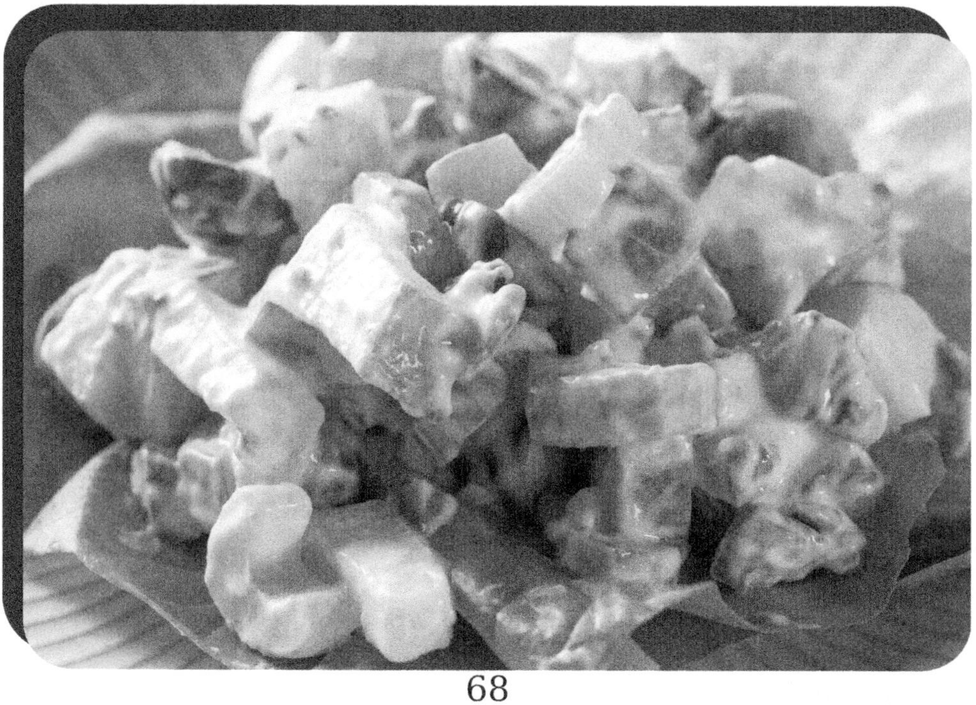

Barbecue Salad

SERVES 4

- 2 large potatoes, cut into thin wedges
- ½ sweet potato, chopped into small pieces
- 1 bunch spring carrots, washed
- Leaves from 1 green cabbage
- 1 cup sliced mushrooms
- 2 cups broccoli florets

For the dressing

- 2 tbsp orange juice
- 3 tbsp olive oil
- Pinch of salt
- Pinch of freshly ground black pepper

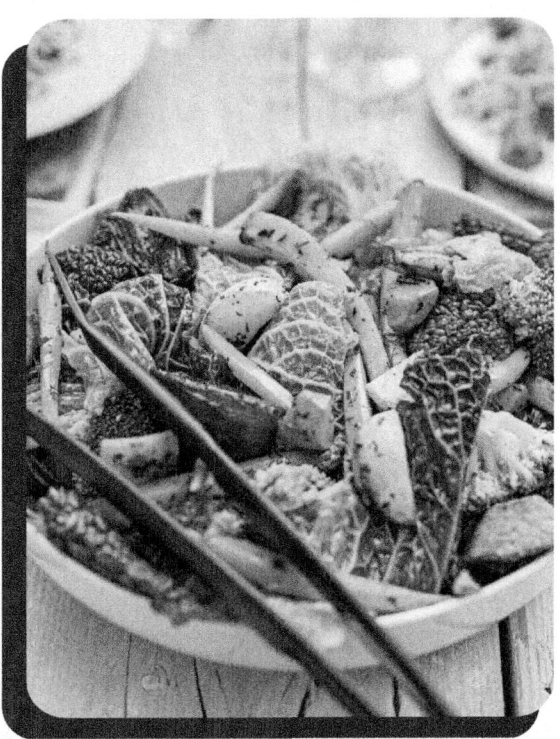

DIRECTIONS

1. Preheat barbecue to medium-high heat.
2. Lightly brush potatoes, sweet potato and carrots with a little oil and place on the barbecue. Cook, turning often for 8-10 minutes or until cooked through and tender. Remove from heat and set aside.
3. Meanwhile add a drizzle of olive oil to a large wok or frying pan and toss in cabbage leaves, mushrooms, and broccoli. Cook, stirring frequently until the broccoli is slightly tender but still has some firmness.
4. Place cabbage, mushrooms, and broccoli in a large serving bowl. Arrange potatoes, sweet potato and carrots on top.
5. Combine orange juice, olive oil, salt and pepper in a small bowl and whisk to combine. Pour dressing over salad and serve.

Raw Carrot Salad

SERVES 4

- 6 large carrots, washed and peeled.
- ¼ cup apple cider vinegar
- 2 tbsp olive oil
- 2 tbsp orange juice
- 1 tsp wholegrain mustard
- 1 tbsp maple syrup
- Salt, to taste
- Freshly ground black pepper, to taste
- 1 ½ cups walnuts

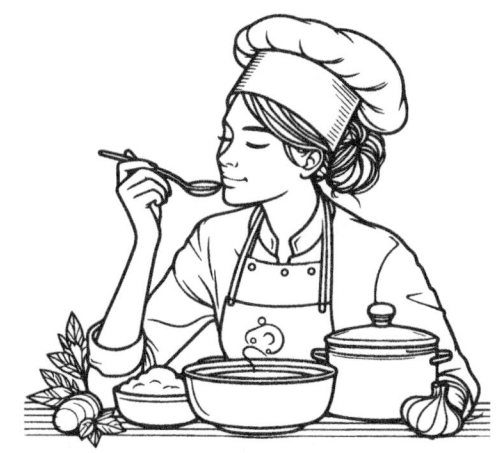

DIRECTIONS

1. Use a vegetable peeler to cut the carrots into ribbons and add to a large bowl.
2. In a small bowl or jug combine apple cider vinegar, olive oil, orange juice, mustard, and maple syrup and whisk well. Season to taste.
3. Pour dressing over carrots and toss to coat. Sprinkle with walnuts and serve.

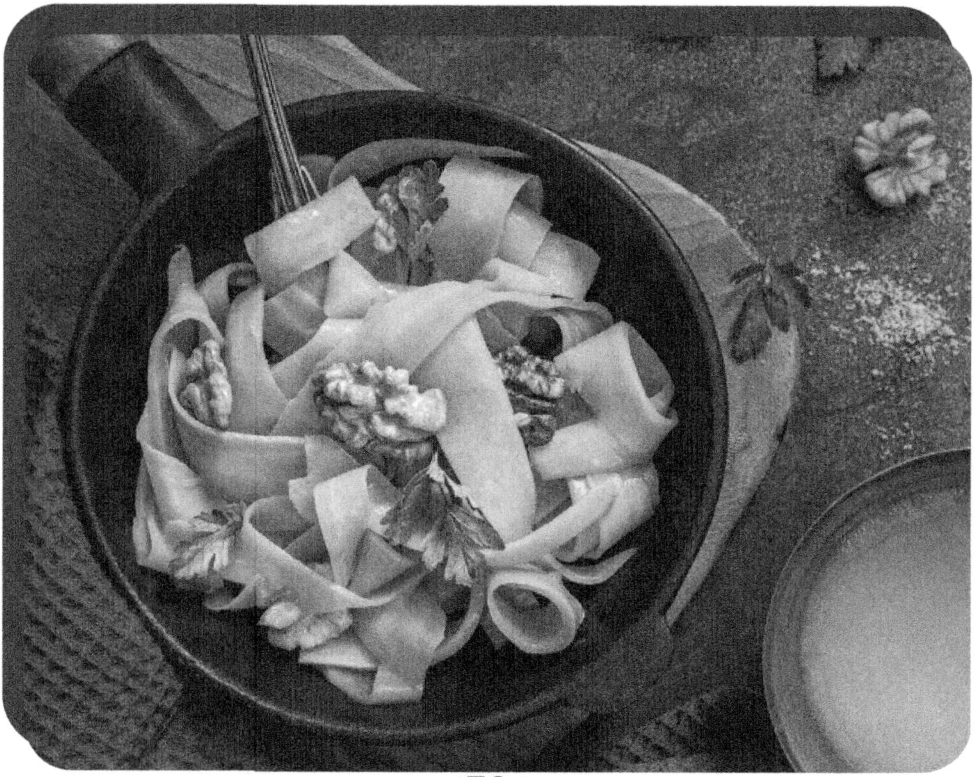

Barbecued Vegetable Rolls

MAKES 12 ROLLS

- 1 red capsicum
- 1 yellow capsicum
- 1 large carrot
- 1 bunch asparagus
- 1 large zucchini
- Salt, to taste
- Freshly ground black pepper, to taste
- ¼ cup olive oil

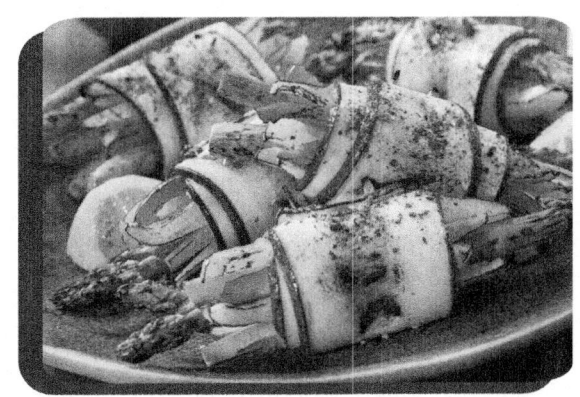

DIRECTIONS

1. Soak 12 toothpicks in water for 15 minutes.
2. Preheat barbecue grill to medium heat.
3. Cut capsicums into strips approximately 6-centimetres long and 1-centimetre wide strip. Peel carrots and cut into pieces the same length as the capsicum. Cut asparagus to the same length.
4. Use a mandolin to slice zucchini into thin ribbons.
5. Lay a zucchini strip on a clean work surface. Season with salt and pepper on both sides. Arrange some capsicum, carrots, and asparagus at one end of the zucchini strip and roll up. Secure with a toothpick. Repeat with remaining zucchini and vegetables have been used.
6. Brush prepared rolls with a little olive oil, reserving some oil for the barbecue.
7. Brush barbecue grill with oil, then place rolls on the barbecue and cook for 10 minutes, turning regularly. When vegetables are softened and the zucchini is charred, remove from barbecue and serve.

TOP TIPS:

- Be sure you soak wooden toothpicks before barbecuing otherwise they will burn.
- Make a quick and easy dressing to go with these rolls by combining 1 cup Greek yoghurt, the juice of half a lemon, 1 clove of minced garlic, and a tablespoon of freshly chopped mint leaves. Mix well and add a little water if you want to have a runnier consistency.

Oi Muchim (Korean Cucumber Salad)

SERVES 4

- 500 g cucumber, sliced
- 1 tsp salt
- 1 clove garlic, minced
- 1 tsp soy sauce
- 3 tbsp rice wine vinegar
- 1 tbsp caster sugar
- 1 tbsp sesame oil
- 2 spring onions, thinly sliced
- 1 tsp chilli flakes (add more if you prefer more spice)
- 2 tbsp toasted sesame seeds

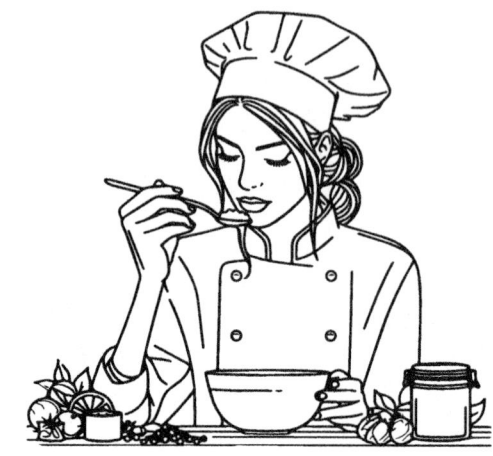

DIRECTIONS

1. Add chopped cucumber to a colander and sprinkle with salt. Set aside to drain for 30 minutes. This will help the cucumbers release water to make the salad crisper.
2. Add garlic, soy sauce, rice wine vinegar, sugar, and sesame oil, to a large bowl and whisk to combine.
3. Rinse cucumber slices and pat dry with paper towel. Add cucumber, spring onions, chilli flakes, and half the sesame seeds to the bowl and toss to coat.
4. Spoon onto a serving plate and scatter with remaining sesame seeds, then serve.

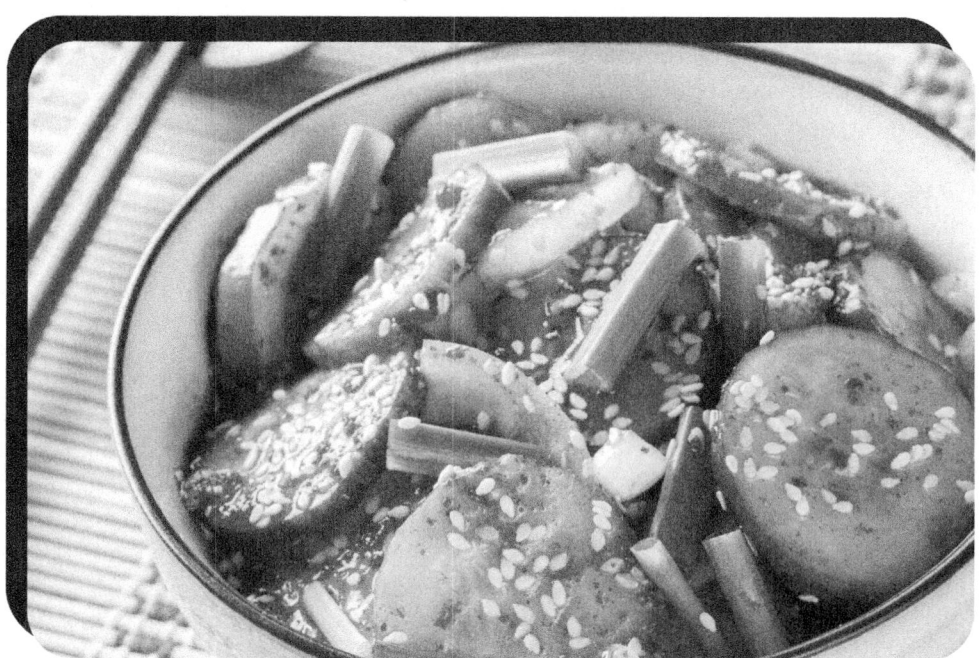

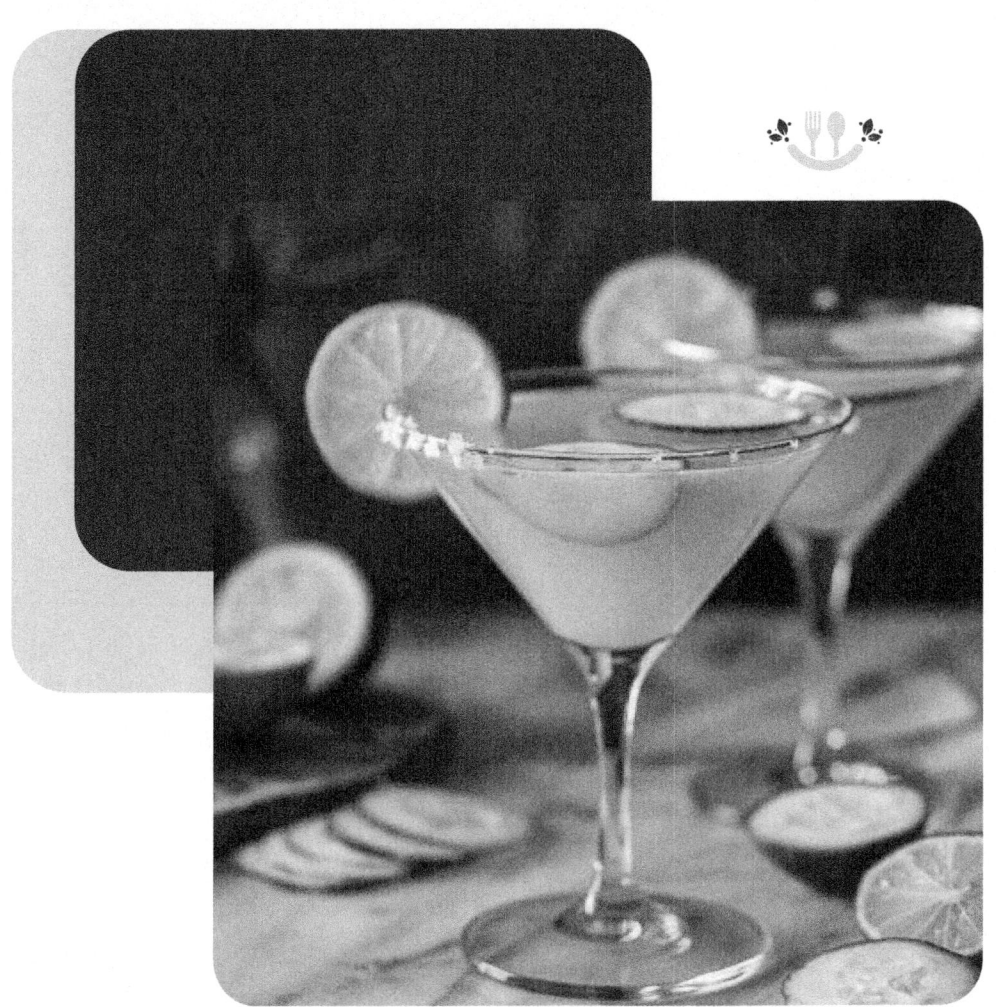

Dink

Drink is a beverage, including any type of liquid that humans can drink. Drinks can be divided into two main categories: alcoholic drinks and non-alcoholic drinks.
Alcoholic beverages: Includes beer, wine, and other spirits. They contain ethanol, an alcohol produced through fermentation and distillation.
Non-alcoholic beverages: Including water, juice, coffee, tea, and many other drinks such as soda, smoothies. This beverage does not contain ethanol.

Cucumber lime martini

SERVES 1

- 60ml vodka or cucumber vodka
- 30ml triple sec
- 1 lime, freshly squeezed
- 1 cup ice
- 2 cucumber slices
- 2 sprigs fresh mint

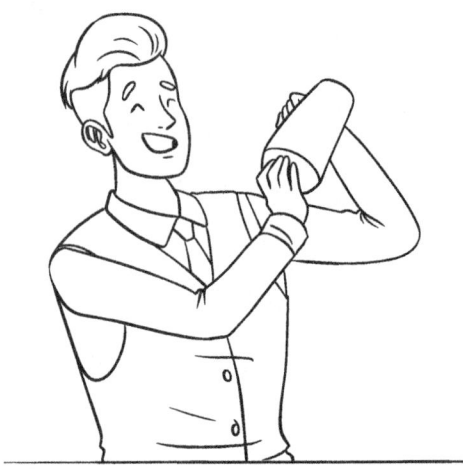

DIRECTIONS

1. Pour vodka, triple sec and lime juice in a cocktail shaker with ice and shake vigorously.
2. Pour into a martini glass and garnish with cucumber slices and mint.

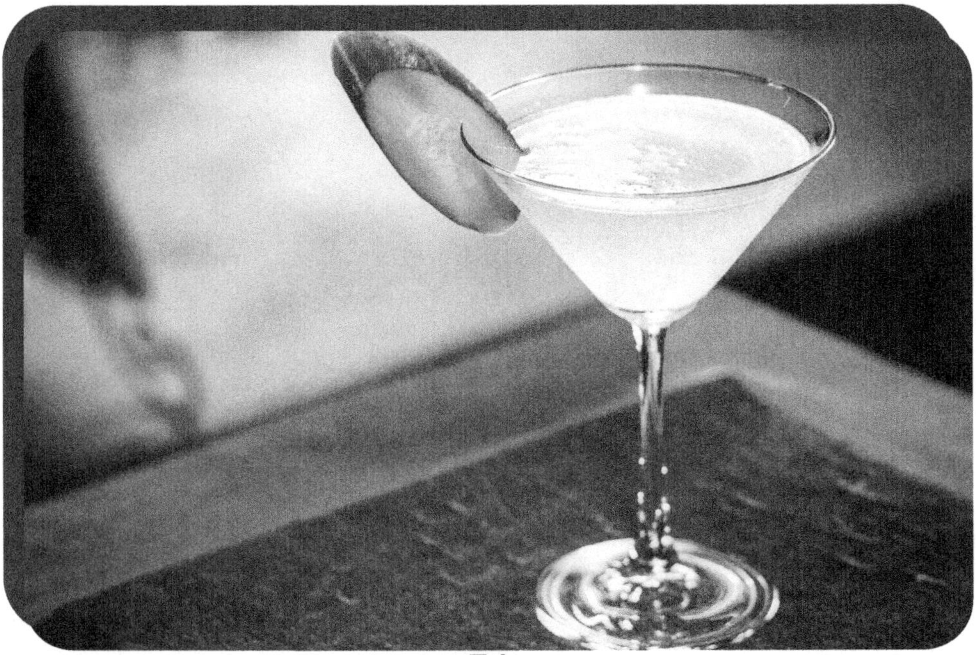

Summer White Sangria

MAKES 6 TO 8 SERVES

- 700g raspberries
- 3 peaches, thinly sliced
- 2 lemons, zest and juice 1 lemon and cut the other into rounds for garnish
- ½ cup orange flavoured liqueur (such as Cointreau)
- ¼ cup peach juice
- 1 ½ bottles white wine, chilled

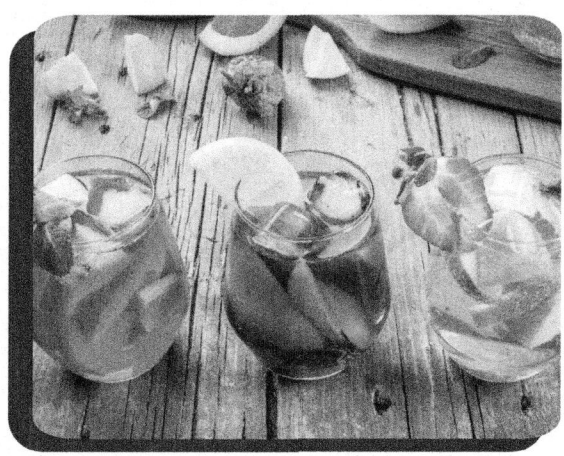

DIRECTIONS

1. Place the peaches and raspberries on a baking tray in an even layer.
2. Put in the freezer for at least 45 minutes or until the fruit is frozen solid. Freezing the fruit means that your sangria will become more flavourful as it chills and the drink won't be diluted by ice cubes.
3. Place the frozen fruit in a large jug. Add lemon zest, lemon juice, peach juice, orange liqueur and wine and stir to combine.
4. Pour into glasses to serve and garnish with lemon.

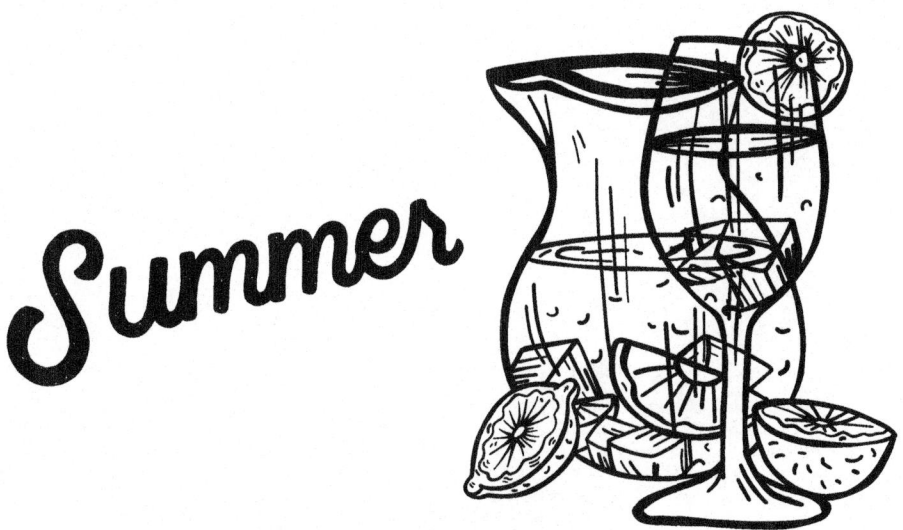

Rosemary and Grapefruit Mimosa

MAKES 8

- 1 cup water
- 1 cup sugar
- 3 fresh rosemary sprigs, plus extra sprigs (small) to garnish
- 750ml sparkling wine, chilled
- 2 cups fresh grapefruit juice
- 1 grapefruit, cut into wedges for garnish

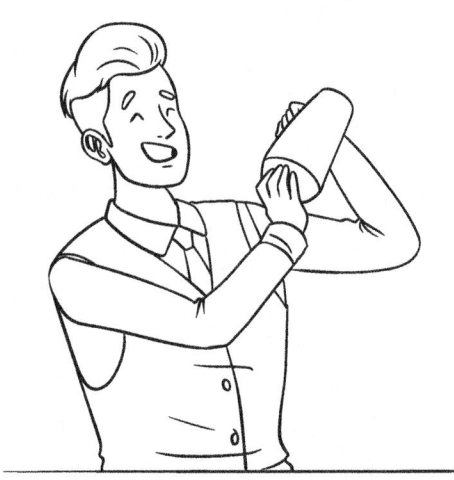

DIRECTIONS

1. Make a rosemary syrup by bringing water and sugar to a simmer in a small saucepan over medium heat. Add the rosemary sprigs and stir into the sugar and water. Remove the saucepan from the heat and cover with a lid. Set aside to steep for 15-20 minutes. Remove the rosemary sprigs from the syrup.
2. To serve, fill eight glasses nearly half full with sparkling wine. Pour ¼ cup grapefruit juice into each lass and add 2 teaspoons of the rosemary syrup. Add a splash more champagne to the glass. Garnish with small rosemary sprigs and wedges of grapefruit.

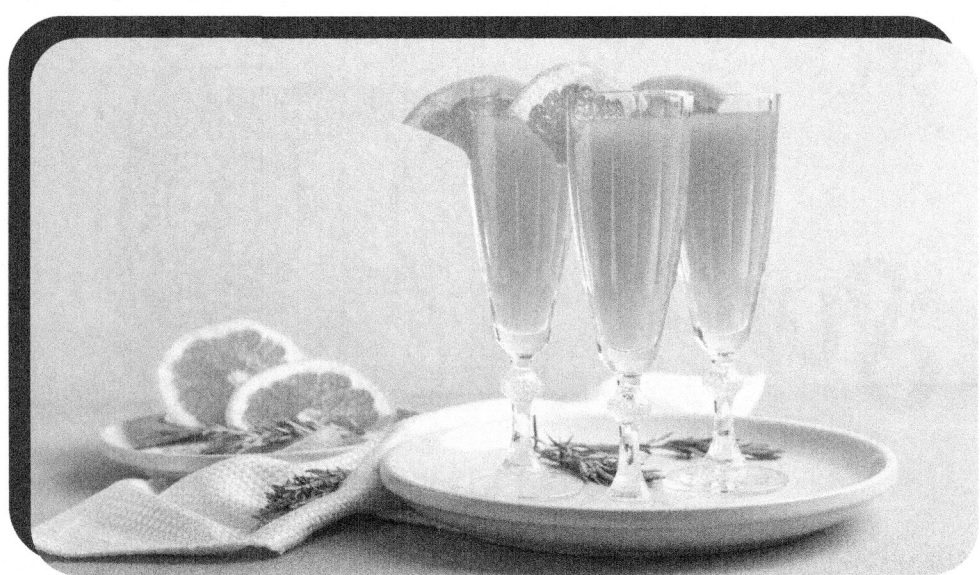

Blood orange cocktail

MAKES 2 ½ CUPS

Blood orange-mint syrup
- 3 cups freshly squeezed blood orange juice (about 12 large oranges)
- 1 cup sugar
- 2 tablespoons chopped fresh mint

Red gin spritz
- 1 shot gin
- 2 shots Blood Orange-Mint Syrup
- Splash of sparkling wine

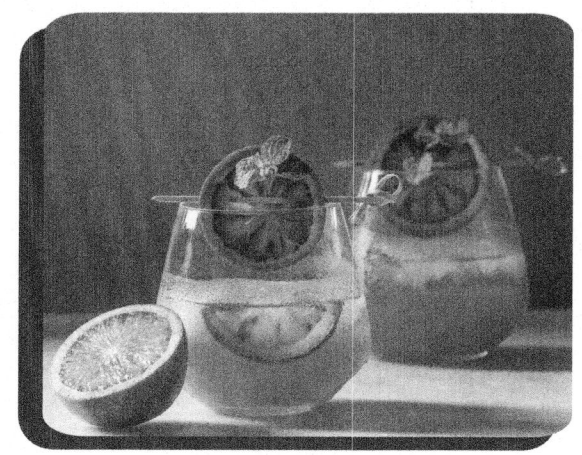

DIRECTIONS

1. Make the syrup: In a medium saucepan, bring the blood orange juice to a boil. Simmer the juice until it has reduced to about 1 cup, 5 to 6 minutes.
2. Add the sugar and return the mixture to a boil, stirring gently to dissolve the sugar. When the sugar is fully dissolved, remove the saucepan from the heat. Stir in the mint. Cool to room temperature.
3. Make the cocktail: In a cocktail shaker filled with ice, shake the gin with the syrup. Strain into a glass and finish with a healthy splash of sparkling wine. Store leftover syrup in the refrigerator for up to two weeks.

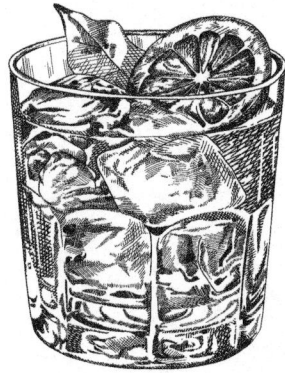
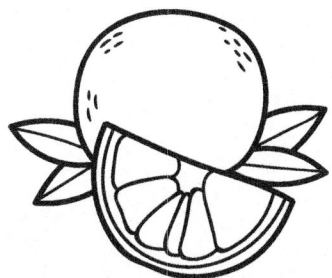

Shaken Strawberry Daiquiri

SERVES 1

- What do I need?
- 30ml fresh lime juice
- 60ml white rum
- 15 ml sugar syrup – see below for how to make this.
- 6 fresh strawberries

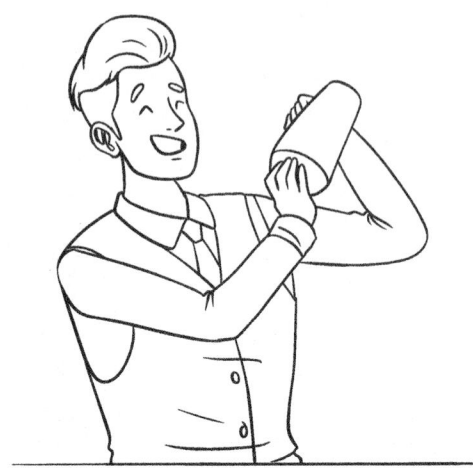

DIRECTIONS

1. To make the sugar syrup combine equal parts sugar and water in a saucepan and bring to a boil. Turn heat down and simmer until sugar dissolves completely and the mixture is clear. Allow to cool and then refrigerate to keep cold.
2. Muddle strawberries in a cocktail shaker.
3. Fill the shaker with ice and add the remaining ingredients.
4. Shake and strain into a chilled martini glass.
5. Garnish with a strawberry.

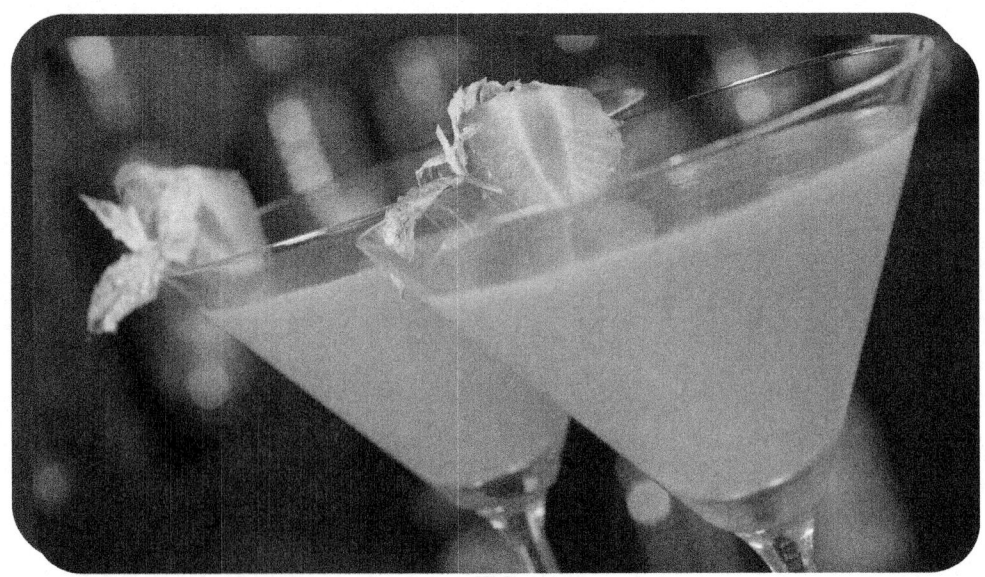

Peanut butter & nutella hot chocolate

MAKES 2 ½ CUPS

- 4 cups low fat or skim milk
- 2 tablespoons Nutella
- 1-2 tablespoons smooth peanut butter
- 2 tablespoons unsweetened cocoa powder
- 2 tablespoons natural sweetener of choice/or raw sugar
- Marshmallows

Optional Toppings:
- Crushed hazelnuts
- Chocolate chips
- Extra Nutella

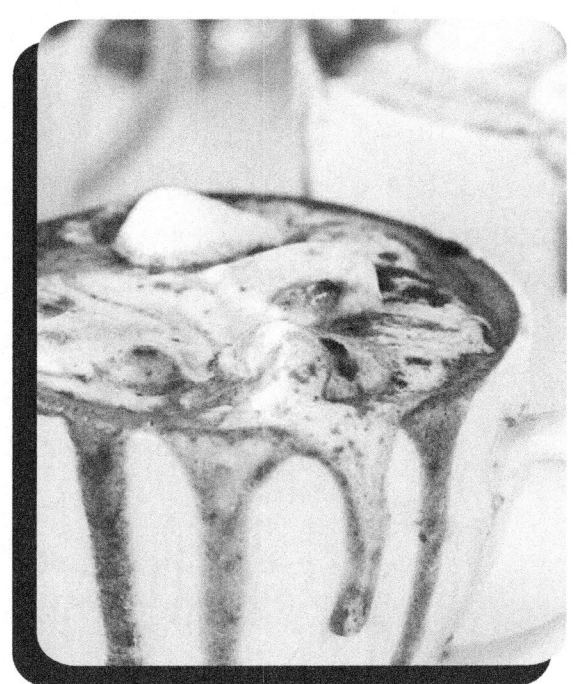

DIRECTIONS

1. Heat milk in a medium sized saucepan on medium to high heat until beginning to warm and steam.
2. Add the Nutella, peanut butter, cocoa powder and sugar, and whisk until dissolved and combined.
3. Bring to a gentle simmer while stirring, and take off heat.
4. Serve with your desired toppings.

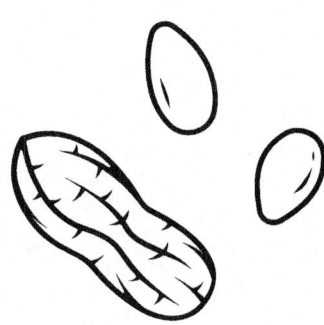

Vegan chai hot chocolate

SERVES 2

- 2 cups vanilla almond milk, sweetened
- 2 tablespoons cocoa powder
- 1 teaspoon Chai Spice

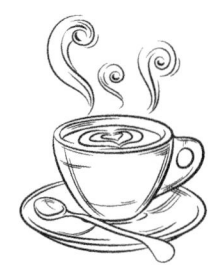

DIRECTIONS

1. Place all ingredients in a medium size sauce pan.
2. Bring to a rolling boil and stir until spices and cocoa powder have dissolved.
3. Reduce heat and let simmer for 3-5 minutes.

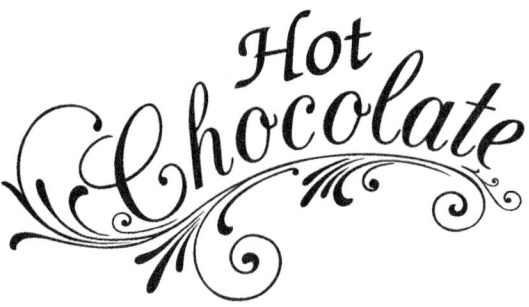

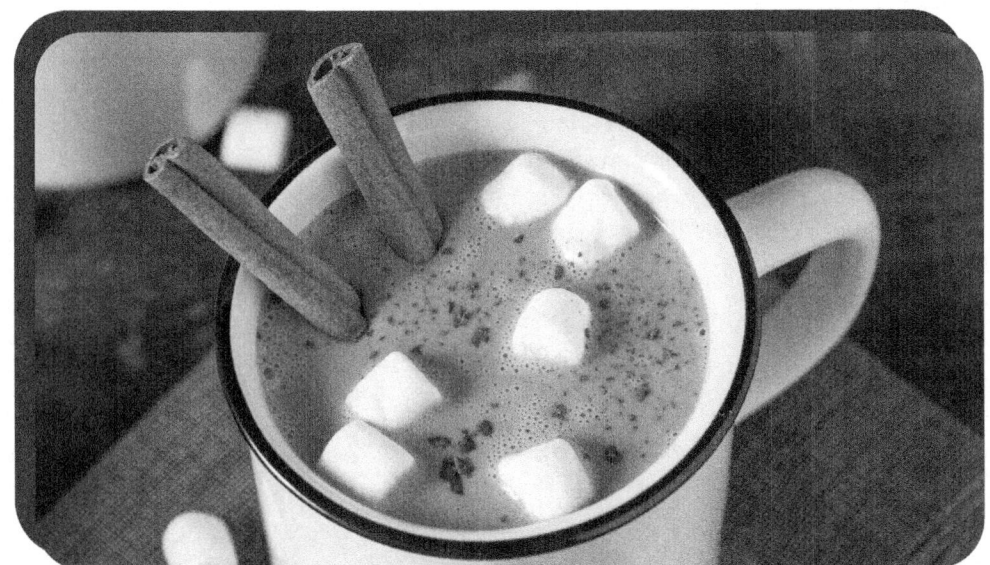

Cheesecake hot chocolate

SERVES 2

- 1 cup milk
- 1/4 teaspoon vanilla extract
- 55g white chocolate, chopped
- 55g cream cheese at room temperature – it is vital that the cream cheese is room temperature because chilled cream cheese will go lumpy. You can use a blender if this happens.
- Sweet biscuit crumbs (eg: Scotch Finger) and whipped cream, for garnish

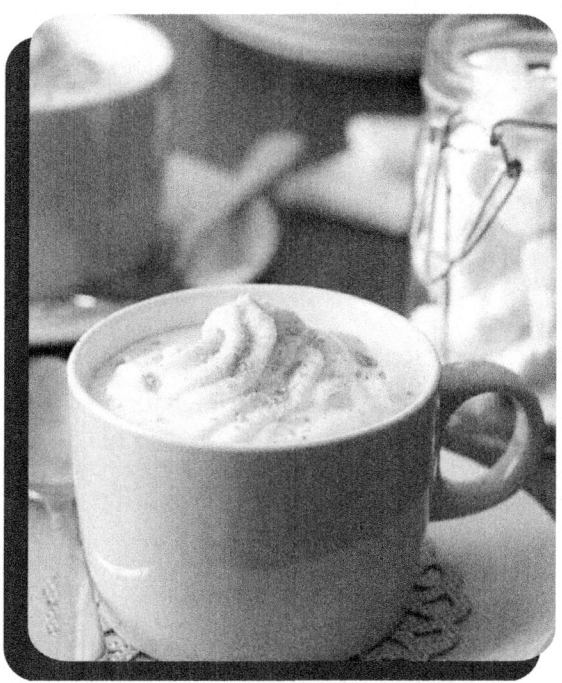

DIRECTIONS

1. In a medium saucepan, warm up the milk over medium heat until hot but not boiling.
2. Turn the heat down to low then whisk in the vanilla and cream cheese until melted.
3. Whisk in the white chocolate until melted and smooth.
4. Serve immediately with whipped cream and biscuit crumbs on top, if desired.

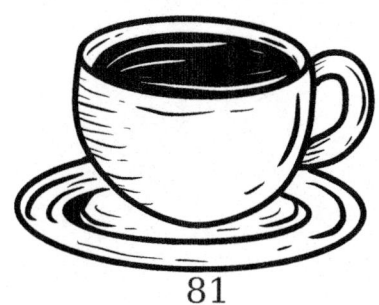

Fresh peach lemonade

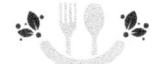

SERVES 5

- 6 fresh peaches, diced
- Zest of 3 lemons
- ½ cup sugar
- 6 cups cold water or sparkling water, divided
- 1 cup fresh lemon juice (juice of about 7 lemons)

For the garnish

- Peach slices
- Lemon slices
- Mint

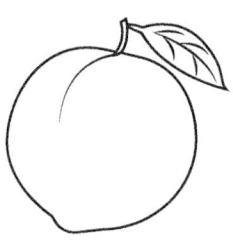

DIRECTIONS

1. In a large saucepan over medium heat, add diced peaches, lemon zest, sugar and 2 cups of water.
2. Stir to dissolve sugar and let mixture simmer - do not boil, reduce heat if needed
3. When peaches are very soft, mash them with a potato masher or fork to break them up.
4. Let mixture simmer until it thickens slightly.
5. Remove from heat and let cool.
6. Strain the peach syrup mixture into a bowl and discard the solids. Allow to cool.
7. Add the lemon juice to the peach mixture.
8. Pour into a jug along with 4 cups of water or sparkling water.
9. Refrigerate until cold.
10. Fill glasses with ice and pour over peach lemonade.
11. Garnish with fresh peach slices, fresh lemon slices and mint.
12. Serve immediately

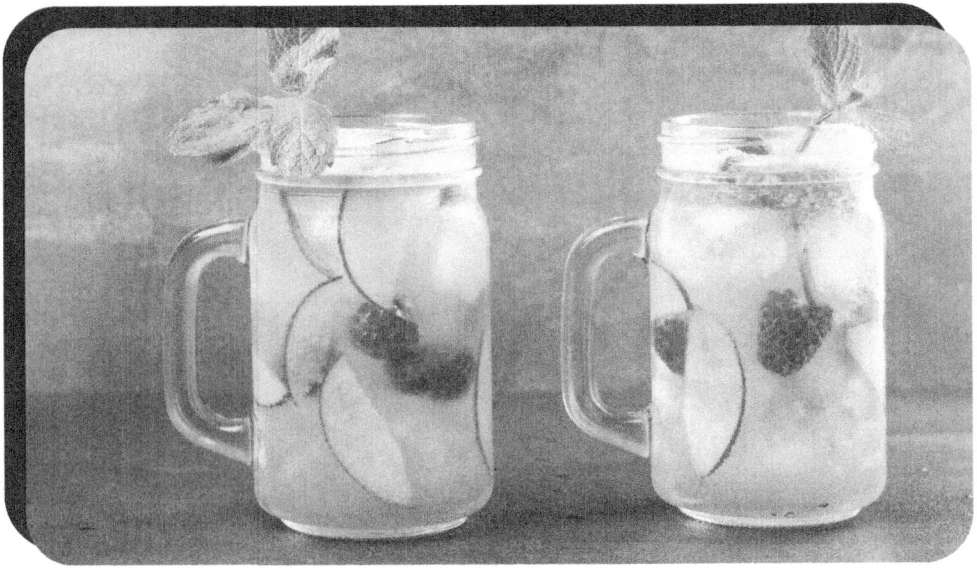

Gin Cocktail

MAKES 2

- 100ml gin
- 100ml tonic water
- 250ml prosecco
- Ice cubes.
- Lychees to serve

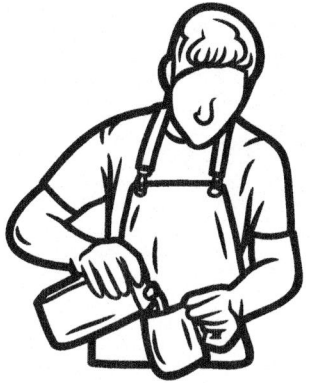

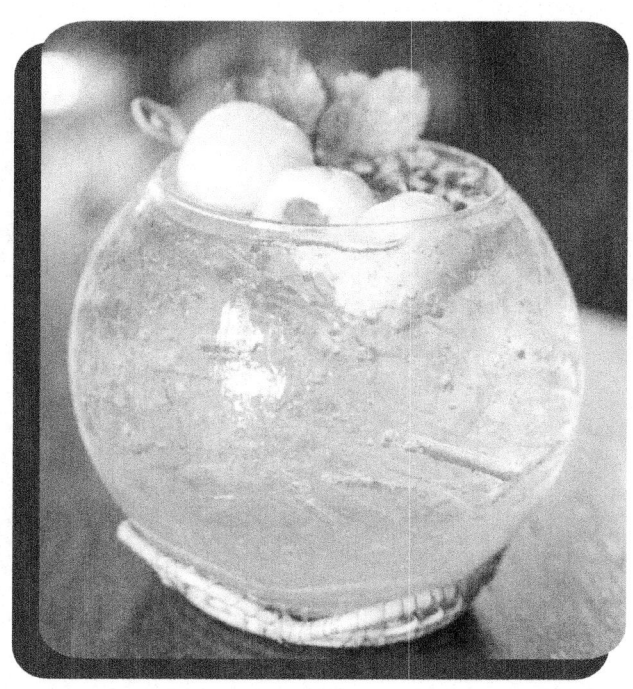

DIRECTIONS

1. Fill 2 glasses with ice cubes.
2. Divide gin and tonic water between the glasses and stir to combine.
3. Top each glass with 125ml prosecco.
4. Garnish with lychees.

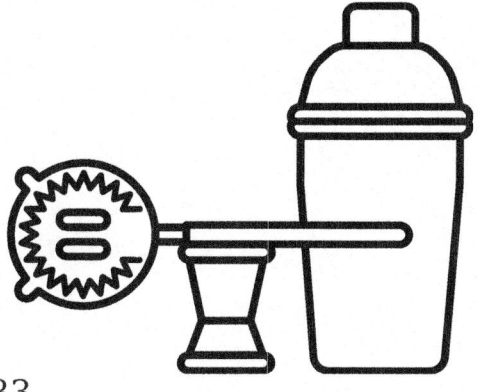

Frozen Watermelon Margaritas

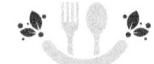

SERVES 4

- 4 cups watermelon, chopped
- ¼ cup lime juice
- ½ cup tequila
- ¼ cup triple sec
- Watermelon wedges for garnish, optional
- Salt for garnish, optional

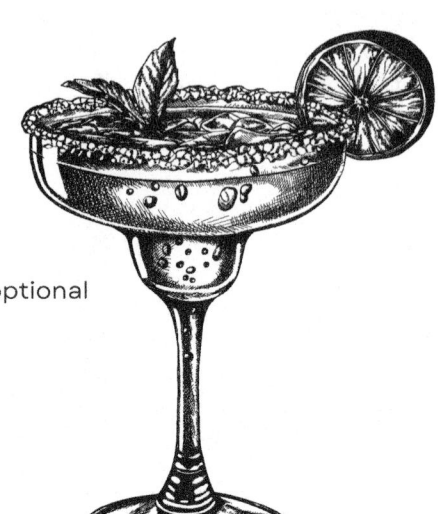

DIRECTIONS

1. Chop watermelon into rough cubes and place in the freezer overnight or for at least 2 hours.
2. Blend frozen watermelon with lime juice, tequila and triple sec until smooth.
3. Pour into glasses and garnish if desired

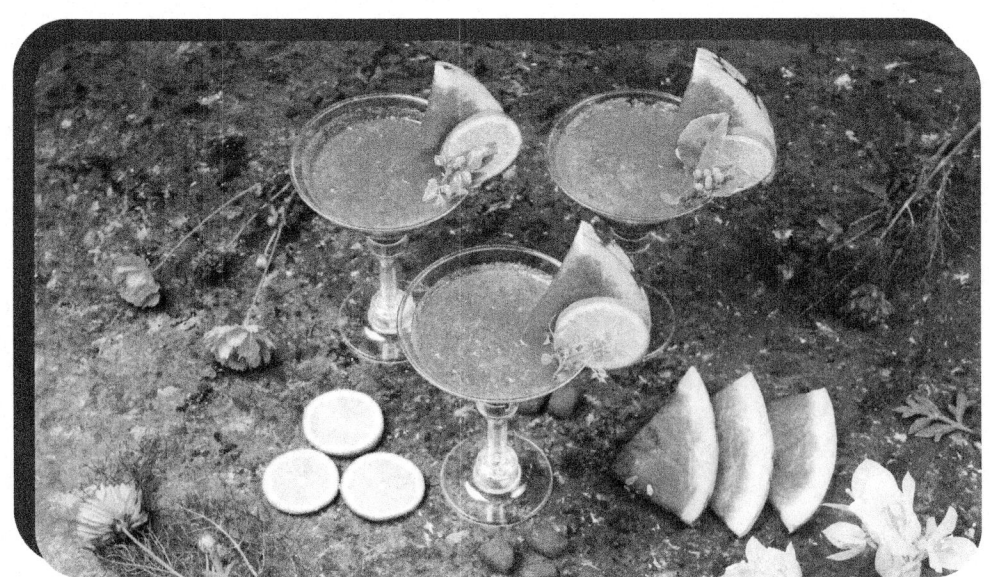

Pine Ginger Mocktail

SERVES 1

- 60 mL pineapple juice
- 8 mint leaves
- Pinch of salt
- 1 tbsp freshly squeezed lime juice
- Ice
- ¾ cup no alcohol ginger beer
- 1 tsp apple cider vinegar
- Pineapple, to garnish

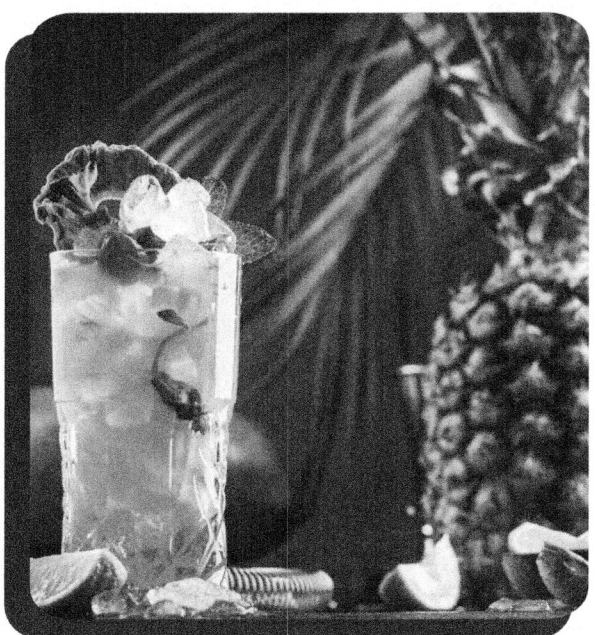

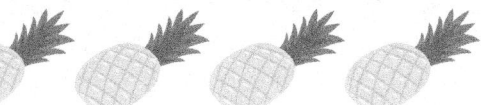

DIRECTIONS

1. Place mint leaves, salt and lime juice into a glass and gently press with a muddler a few times. Add ice to the glass and then pour in pineapple juice and apple cider vinegar and stir.
2. Add ginger beer and garnish with pineapple.

TOP TIP:

3. A muddler is a bar tool designed to smash and mix (muddle) ingredients, much like a pestle. If you don't have a muddler, you can use the handle of a wooden spoon to muddle drinks.

Choc Mint Martini

SERVES 1

- 30 mL vanilla vodka
- 30 mL chocolate syrup
- 30 mL Crème de Menthe
- 45 mL milk
- Ice cubes
- Whipped cream, to garnish
- Grated chocolate, to garnish

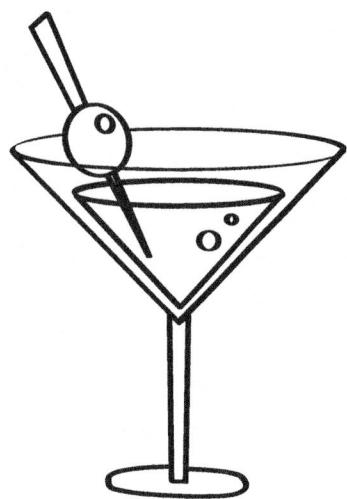

DIRECTIONS

1. Add vodka, chocolate syrup, Crème de Menthe, and milk to a cocktail shaker filled with ice. Shake well and strain into a cocktail glass.
2. Garnish with a dollop of whipped cream and grated chocolate.

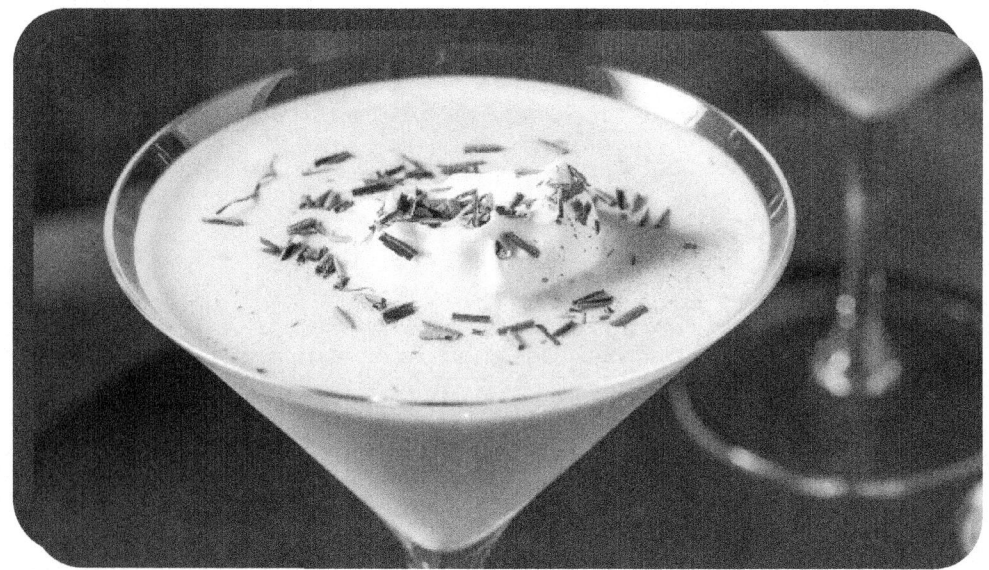

Salted Caramel Kahlua Cream

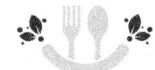

SERVES 1

- 1 tbsp caramel sauce or syrup, plus extra to drizzle
- 60 mL vodka
- 30 mL Kahlua
- 30 mL thickened cream
- Ice cubes
- Sea salt, to garnish

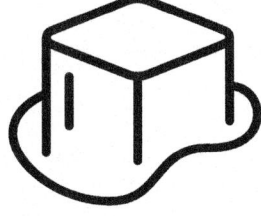

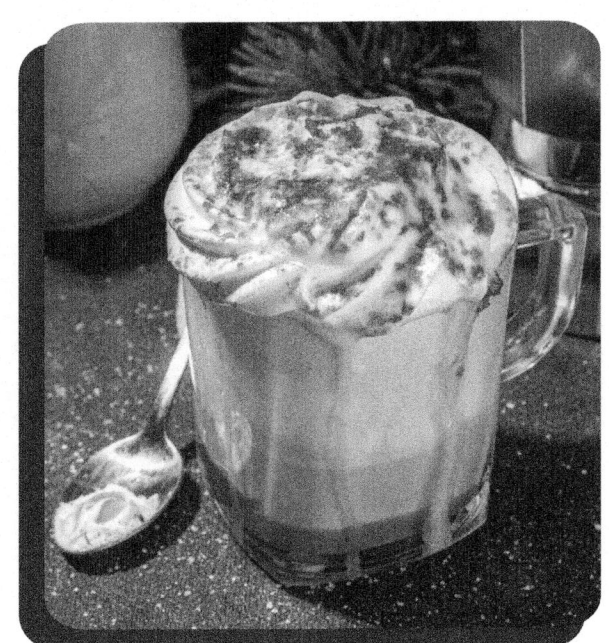

DIRECTIONS

1. Prepare cocktail glass by pouring a little caramel sauce onto a small plate and some sea salt onto a separate plate. Dip rim of glass in the sauce and then dip it in the salt. Set aside.
2. Add 1 tbsp caramel sauce, vodka, Kahlua and cream to cocktail shaker with a handful of ice cubes. Shake vigorously, then strain into glass.
3. Drizzle with a little extra caramel sauce and serve.

Peppermint Mimosas with Candy Canes

SERVES 6

- 180 mL peppermint vodka, divided
- 1 bottle prosecco
- 7 candy canes

DIRECTIONS

1. Crush 1 candy cane into small pieces. Transfer to a plate. Wet the rim of 6 champagne flutes and roll in the crushed candy cane.
2. Add 30 mL peppermint vodka to each glass. Top with prosecco. Garnish with a whole candy cane.

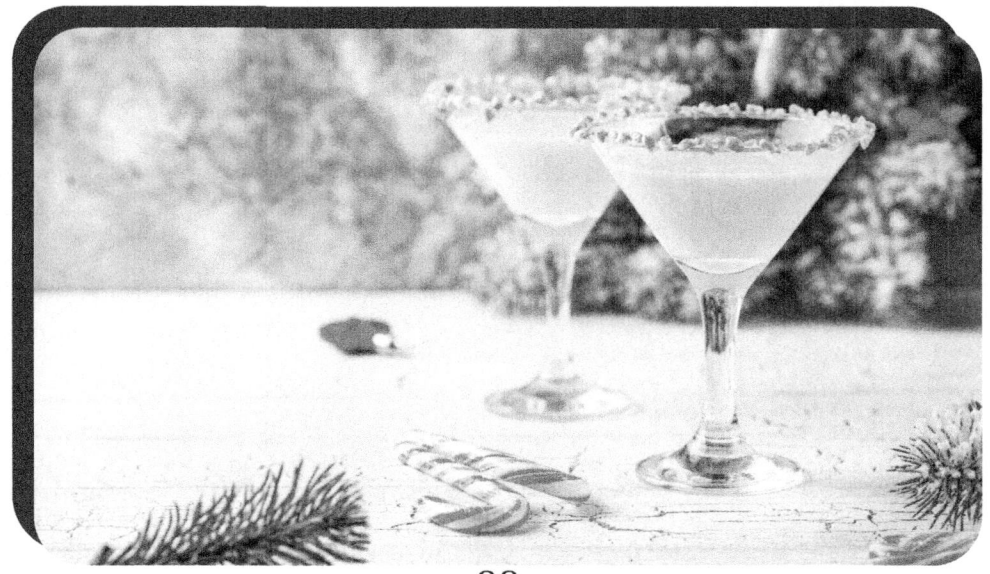

Bloody Mary

SERVES 2

- 2 cups ice cubes
- 100 mL vodka
- 500 mL tomato juice
- 1 tbsp lemon juice
- Tabasco Sauce to taste
- 4 dashes Worcestershire sauce
- Salt and pepper to taste
- 2 celery sticks
- 2 stuffed green olives
- Lime slices to garnish

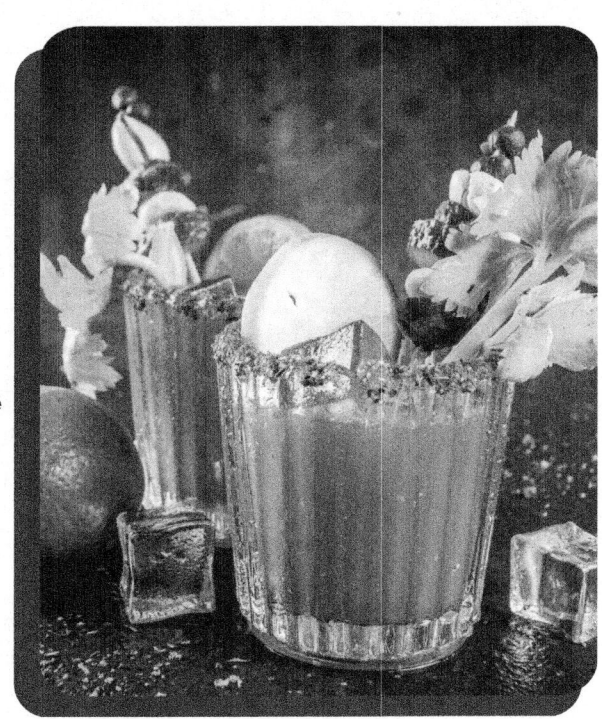

DIRECTIONS

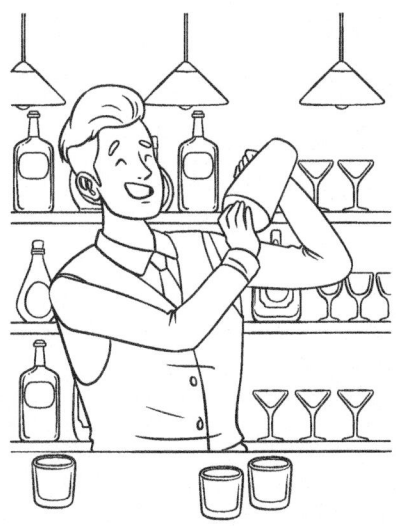

1. Place ice in a large jug. Add vodka, tomato juice, lemon juice, Worcestershire sauce, Tabasco and salt and pepper. Stir well and strain into 2 glasses.
2. Top up with extra ice. Place olives on a toothpick or mini skewer. Garnish with a stick of celery, a slice of lime and the olives.

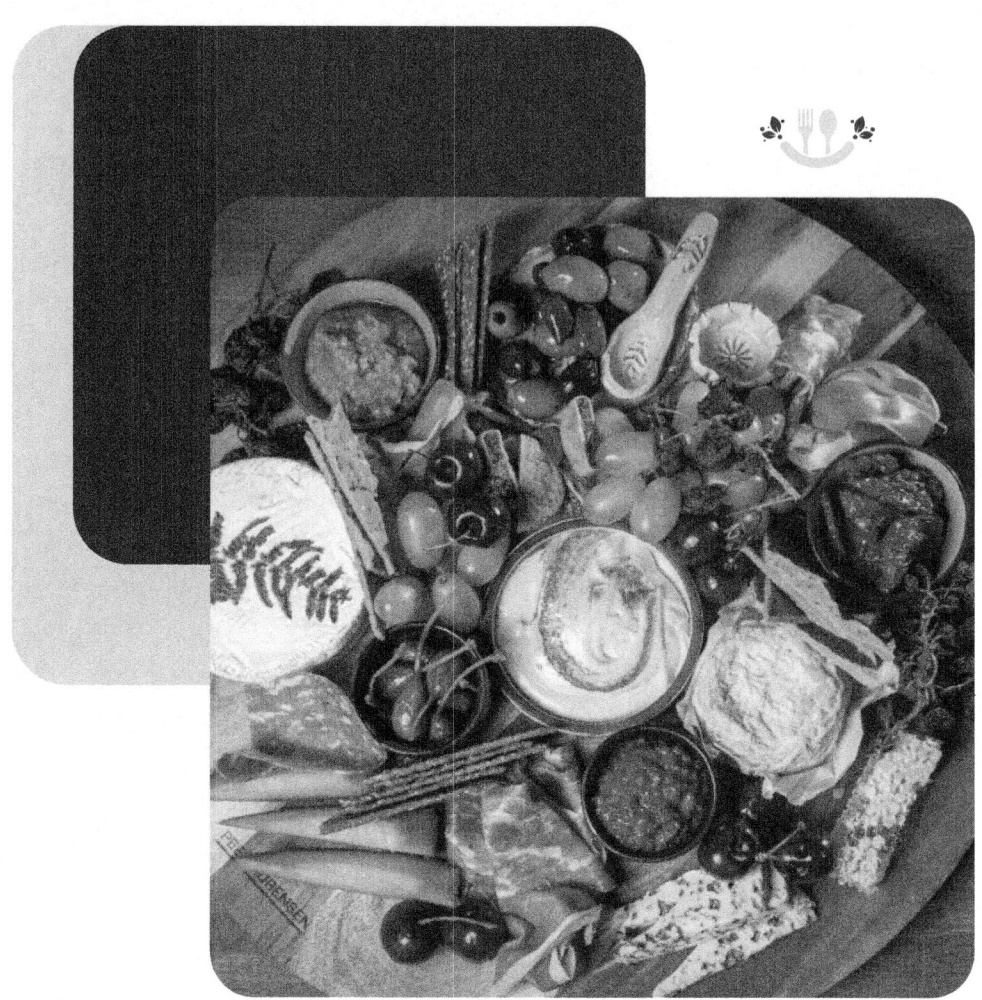

Dressings, Sauces and Jams

"Dressings, Sauces, and Jams" are three different types of culinary products:

Dressings: Dressings are mainly used to dress salads, usually made from oil, vinegar, spices and herbs, helping to enhance flavor and soften salad ingredients.

Sauces: Liquid or thick mixtures used to add flavor or moisture to dishes, which may or may not be cooked, and are used in the preparation or presentation of dishes.

Jams: A product of crushed or chopped fruit and sugar, often with pectin added to help thicken during cooking, used to preserve fruit and often applied to bread or used in baking recipes.

Comice pear and apple chutney

- 1.5kg Comice pears, peeled, cored and diced into 3 centimetre pieces
- 1kg Granny Smith apples, peeled, cored and diced into 3 centimetre pieces
- 2 cups pomegranate juice
- 4 cups apple cider vinegar
- 2 cups of sugar
- ½ red onion diced
- ½ cup sour cherries
- 10 centimetre piece of ginger- grated
- 2 red chillis seeded & diced
- 1 star anise
- Salt & Pepper to taste

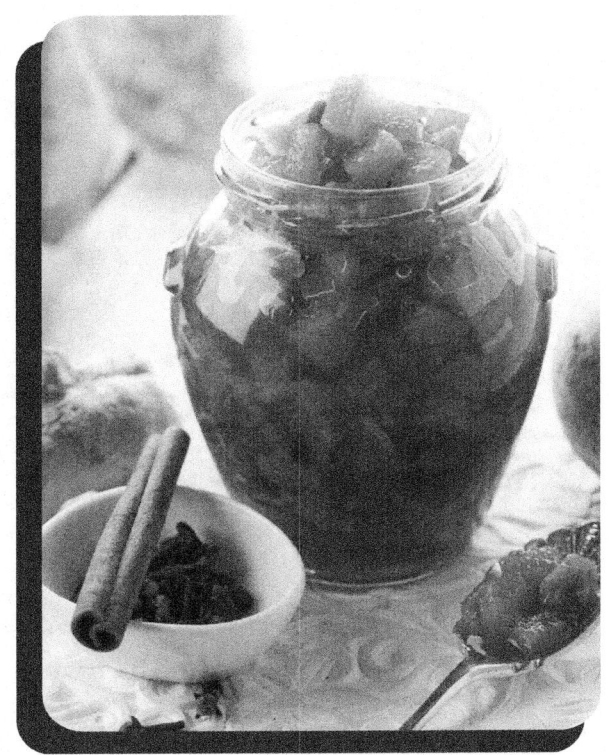

DIRECTIONS

1. Bring pomegranate juice, vinegar, sugar and star anise to a boil in a large stockpot.
2. Reduce heat to medium high and cook until liquid is reduced to 2 ½ - 3 cups. It should be rather thick and syrupy.
3. Add the pears, apples, ginger, chilli, onion, and cherries and cook until the fruit is soft- about 30 minutes.
4. Lower heat and cook down further until the liquid is very thick
5. Remove from heat and let rest for about 30 minutes before spooning into sterilised jars
6. Enjoy this chutney with brie, on sandwiches, with roast pork or with basmati rice and naan.

Quick tomato chutney

- 250g finely sliced red onions
- 500g mixed tomatoes, roughly chopped
- 1 red chilli, deseeded and sliced
- 75ml red wine vinegar
- 140g brown sugar

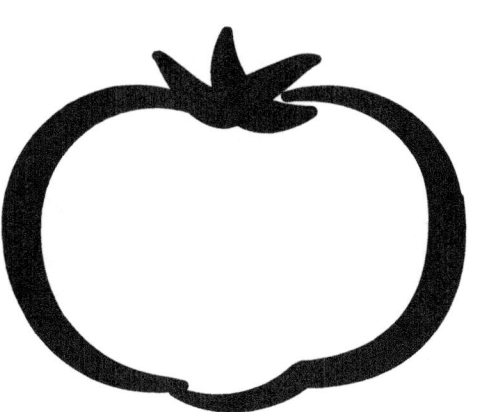

DIRECTIONS

1. Put everything in a pan, season to taste with salt and pepper and stir well to combine.
2. Simmer on the stove for 30-40 minutes or until jammy.
3. Pour into sterilised jars and leave to cool before transferring to the fridge or pantry.

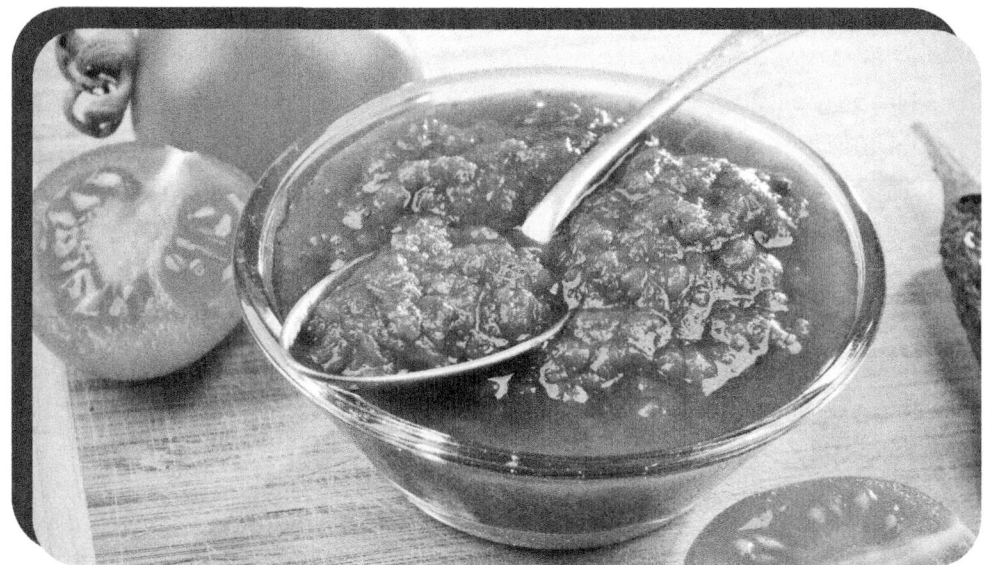

Fresh peach chutney

- 1kg yellow peaches, peeled
- 1 small red onion, finely chopped
- 2 garlic cloves, crushed
- 5cm piece of fresh ginger, peeled and grated
- 1/2 cup malt vinegar
- 1/2 cup white sugar
- 2 tbs sweet chilli sauce

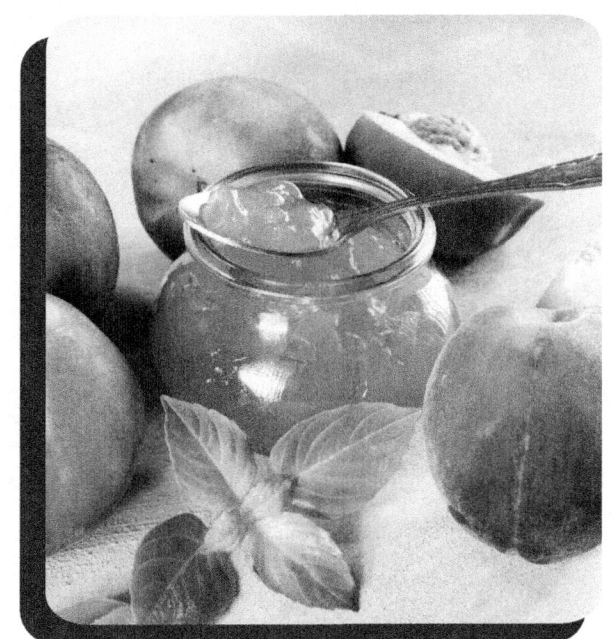

DIRECTIONS

1. Cut the peaches in half. Remove the stones and roughly chop the flesh.
2. Combine peaches, onion, garlic, ginger, vinegar, sugar and sweet chilli in a 3 litre capacity saucepan. Cook on a low heat for 25-30 minutes or until chutney is thick.
3. Spoon the hot chutney into hot sterilized jars and seal. Refrigerate after opening.
4. Serve with ham or turkey, or use on sandwiches.

Spiced mango chutney

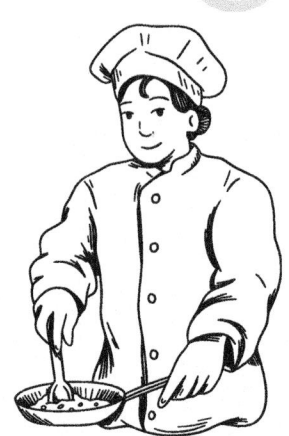

- 1½ tbsp vegetable oil
- 1 Spanish onion, finely chopped
- ½ tsp ground allspice
- 150 ml cider vinegar
- 1/3 cup brown sugar
- 3 firm, ripe mangoes, coarsely chopped

DIRECTIONS

1. Heat oil in a saucepan over medium heat, add onion and stir occasionally until soft and translucent (5-10 minutes).
2. Add allspice and cook until fragrant (10-20 seconds), then add vinegar, sugar and mango and stir occasionally until thick (30-40 minutes).
3. Season to taste, spoon into sterilised jars, seal jars and stand until cooled, then store in refrigerator.

Notes: Mango chutney will keep refrigerated for 2-3 weeks after opening.

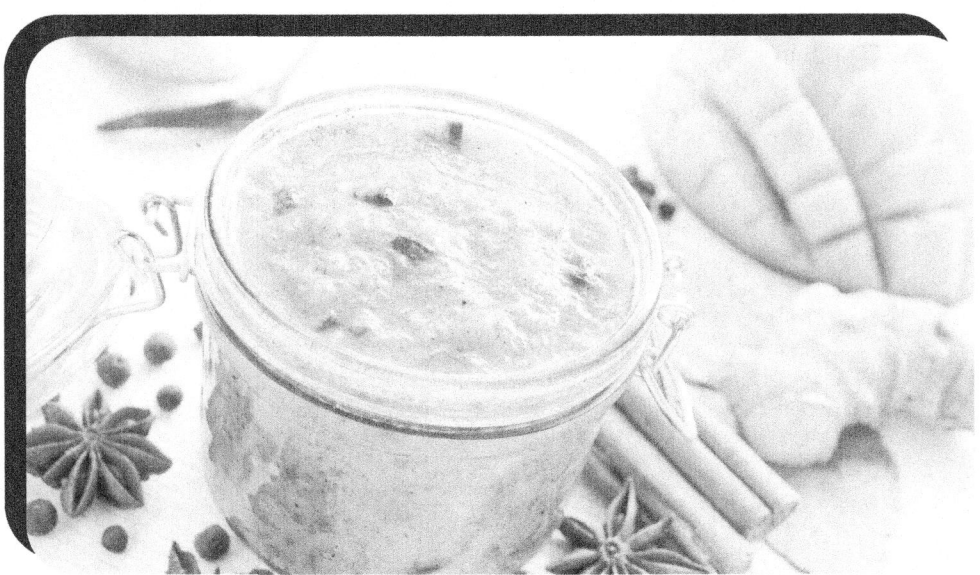

Spicy Mango Dipping Sauce

MAKES APPROXIMATELY 1 CUP OF SAUCE

- 1 tightly packed cup of fresh mango, diced
- 3 tbsp coriander leaves, roughly chopped
- 2 tbsp red onion, finely chopped
- 1 tbsp soy sauce
- 1 tbsp sriracha
- ½ small red chilli, seeds removed, chopped
- 2 ½ tbsp coconut milk
- Salt and pepper to taste

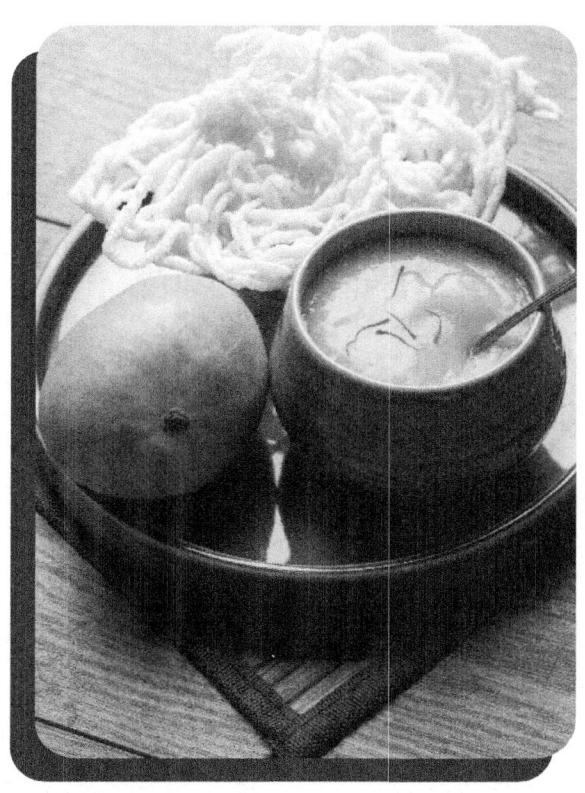

DIRECTIONS

Blitz all ingredients using a stick blender or in a food processor. Taste and season to taste. If the sauce is too thick add extra coconut milk to achieve desired consistency

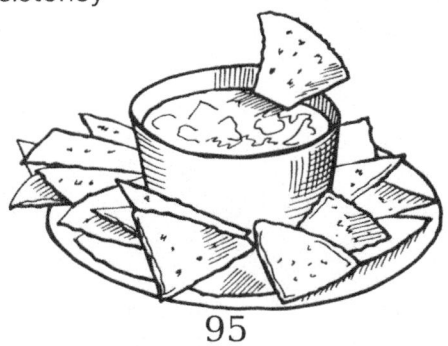

Best ever barbecue sauce

10 MINUTES

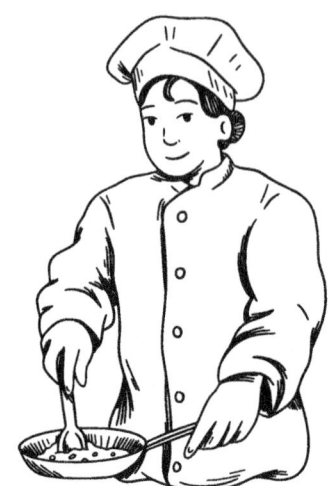

- ½ cup brown sugar
- ¾ cup tomato sauce
- ¼ cup red wine vinegar
- ¼ cup water
- 1 ½ tsp Worcestershire sauce
- 1 tsp paprika
- ½ tsp salt
- ½ tsp freshly ground black pepper
- Tabasco sauce to taste

DIRECTIONS

Blend or whisk together all ingredients until smooth.

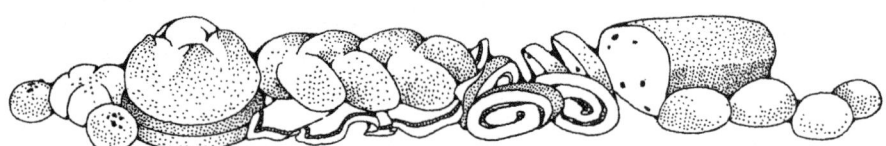

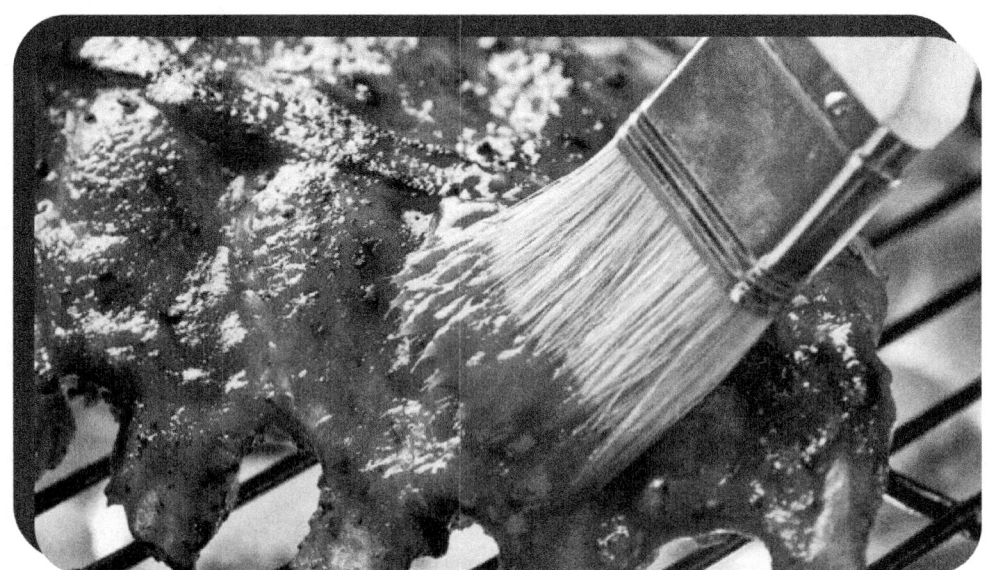

Christmas Marmalade

MAKES APPROXIMATELY 350 GRAMS

- 100g brown sugar
- 500g red onion, thinly sliced
- 30g dried cranberries
- 25ml red wine vinegar
- 50ml port
- 1 tsp dried thyme
- 1 tbsp olive oil

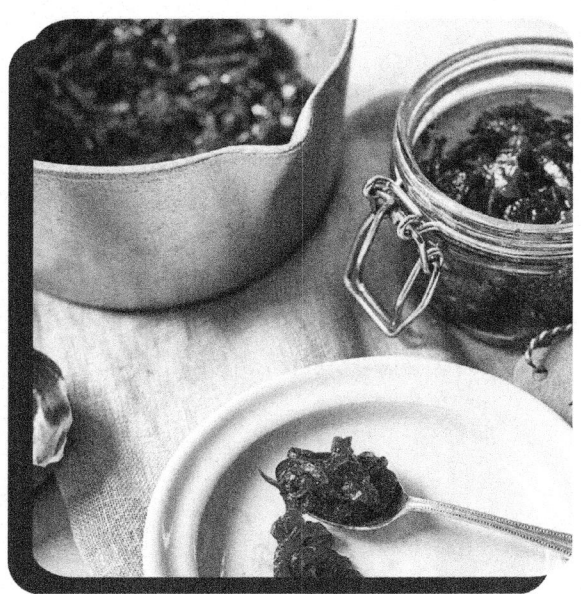

DIRECTIONS

1. Heat oil in large saucepan over medium-low heat. Add onions and a pinch of salt. Cover with a lid and cook for 10 minutes, stirring occasionally.
2. After 10 minutes remove lid, add sugar, thyme and cranberries. Cover with lid and cook for a further 10 minutes.
3. Remove lid and add vinegar and port and turn heat up. Bring to a boil and cook uncovered until the liquid is nearly all evaporated and the onions are very soft. Remove from heat and allow to cool completely.
4. Store marmalade in a sterilised jar in a cool, dark place for up to 6 months. When opened, store in the fridge for up to 1 month.

Beetroot Hummus

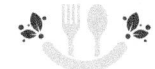

SERVES 10

- 200 g beetroot, chopped
- 400 g tin chickpeas, drained
- 2/3 cup tahini
- 1/3 cup lemon juice
- Zest of 2 lemons
- 2 cloves garlic
- 1/3 cup olive oil
- 1 tsp salt

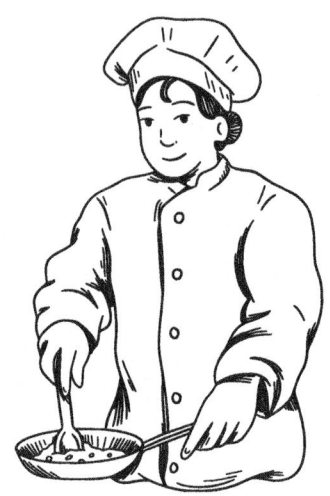

DIRECTIONS

1. Add beetroot, chickpeas, tahini, lemon juice and zest, and garlic to a food processor. With the motor running slowly add olive oil, blending until smooth. Taste and season if needed.
2. Serve with crackers or bread.

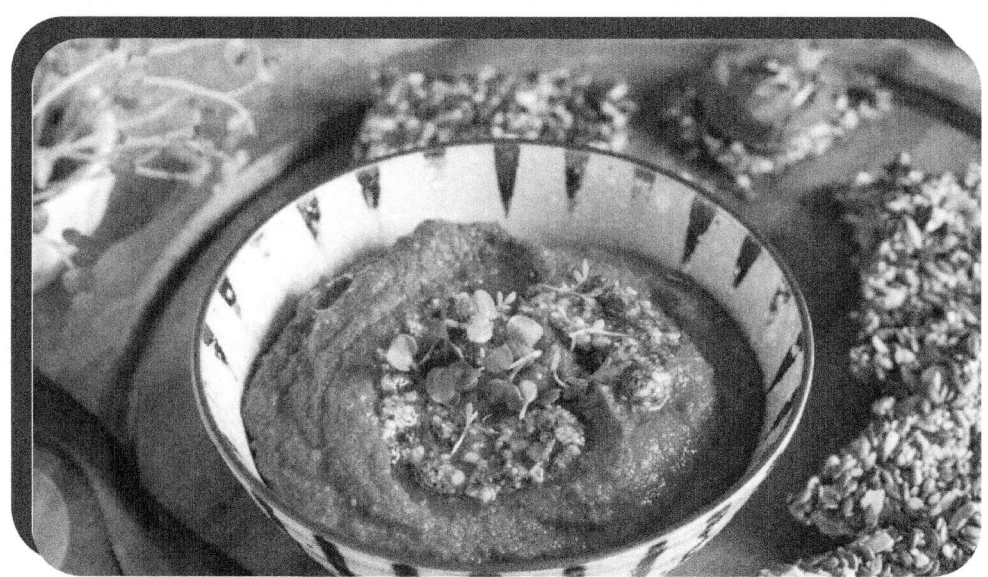

Cranberry Chutney

MAKES APPROXIMATELY 10 SERVINGS

- 1 cup orange juice
- 350 g fresh or frozen cranberries (if using frozen, there is no need to defrost)
- 1 orange, including peel, seeds removed
- 1 Granny Smith apple, cored
- 12 dried apricots
- 1 ¼ cups honey
- Pinch of salt

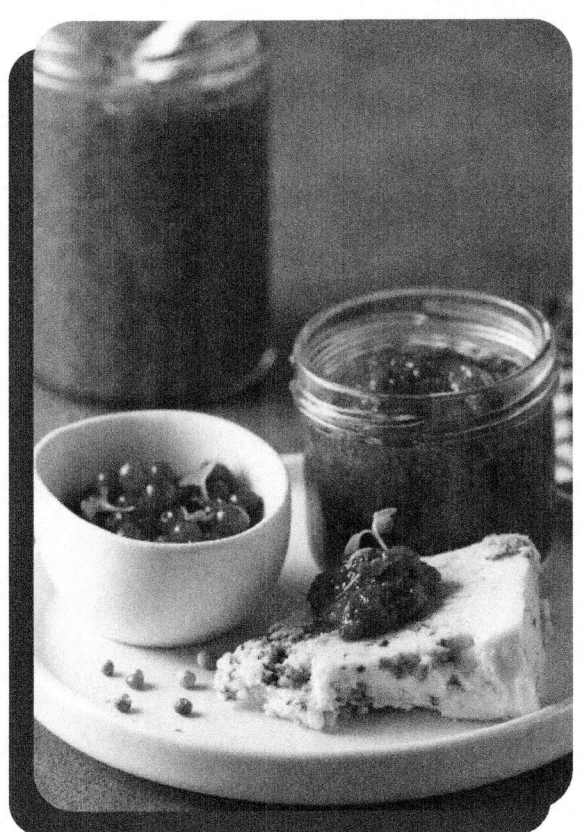

DIRECTIONS

1. Chop orange and apple roughly and place in a saucepan over medium heat with orange juice and cranberries. Bring to the boil and cook over medium heat until the berries start to break down.
2. Add remaining ingredients and cook for a further 10 minutes or until thick. Taste and adjust seasoning if needed.
3. Remove from heat and set aside to cool, then place in a clean jar and use within 1 week.

Heart Healthy
COOKBOOK

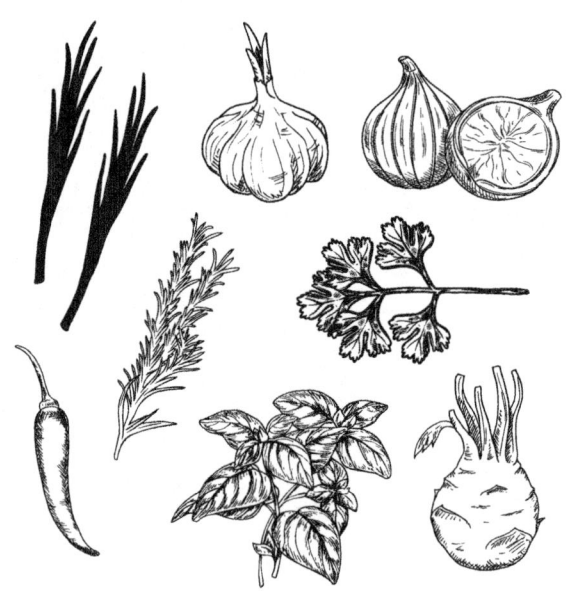

— Thank you —

Printed in Great Britain
by Amazon